POST-PREGNANCY:

EASING INTO FITNESS.

Crystal Watkins

Copyright

Title book: Post-Pregnancy

       Easing Into Fitness

Author book: Crystal Watkins

Dedication....

Karli, Staci, Stedman, Mom, and Dad

Table of Contents

Exercise and Activity

Positive Habits for A Healthy Lifestyle

Women who have recently given birth are likely looking for fast weight loss solutions, and the best methods for weight loss after a new baby. But it is not just about the foods you eat and the exercise you are going to start to include in your daily life. It is also about making positive choices and lifestyle changes, to live a healthier life! You want to lose the weight, but you also should focus on making positive changes and lifestyle habits, in order to raise your child in a healthy home, and in order to ensure you are happy after giving birth to your child. There are certain things you can do in order to create a healthy lifestyle, and these should be followed through not only after giving birth, but also throughout the rest of your life.

Meditate –

Creating a few minutes each day and allowing yourself to clear the mind is something great for new moms to do. Not only is it going to allow you to think clearly, it is also going to give you a fresh start to each new day. You can meditate anywhere; you simply have to find a way to clear your mind, to let go of your stresses and thoughts, and focus on creating a positive image, so you can improve your day, and so you can improve the way you are going to raise your child.

Show thanks –

This does not necessarily mean being religious or praying; instead, it just means being thankful for the things that you have in your life. We often focus on the negative, and all the bad that we encounter. Instead, look at your newborn child, your spouse, and all the good things you have in your life, and be thankful. We should be thankful that we get up every morning, but we generally focus on the bad. Make it a habit to focus on the good, and have thanks for the good things that you have going on for you in your life.

Laughter –

You are quickly going to learn that with a newborn you are going to have plenty of joy, but along with that comes more stress. Not only are you going to miss sleeping, you are also going to be hit with more of a financial burden, and you are responsible for taking care of a new life, in addition to all other worries and stresses in your life. Find a way to laugh each day; whether it is watching a movie or show, talking to a friend, or doing something that makes you happy, this is a great way to eliminate some of the stress you deal with, and it is going to help you clear your mind, so you can be the best parent possible.

Write things down –

Every day you are going to face a setback or a new challenge, especially as a new mom. Keep a journal, and write those down, as well as any progression that you have made. By doing this, you are going to find that it is easy to see where you have to make changes in your life, you are going to find it easier to notice the places that you are struggling, and it is going to allow you to see the good that you are doing as well. By simply writing things down, it is going to be easier for you to modify and make changes where necessary, since you can see where you are struggling, and what you have to do to become a better person and a better parent.

Get a massage –

You need to take time out for you, especially as a new mother. Go out once a month, or even once a week and take a day for you. Get a massage, go to an acupuncture session, or do anything at a spa that makes you happy. This is not only going to help relax you, it is also going to help you feel calm, and help eliminate many of the stresses that you are dealing with in your life. Everyone is different, and everyone deals with stress in a different way; consider taking some time out for you every once in a while, in order for you to recharge, and start over with a fresh mind and body.

Walk –

Get in at least 10,000 steps a day. Even if you are not able to get in a full body workout for the day, or go out to the gym, try to go out to the park and walk with your baby in the stroller. If you can't do this, walk around your home or your building, walk up and down the stairs at work, or do anything to keep you moving. When you move, you are not only going to feel better, you are also going to look better. Additionally, exercise, and getting outside to get some sunshine, is a great way for you to refresh your mind, and look at your day in a completely different way. So, if you are having a bad day, or if you are tired, you can simply go out for a walk, and you are going to find that this is instantly going to enhance your mood, and you are bound to feel better once you get back to the office or once you get back home.

Choose the right foods –

A healthy diet is not only going to help you lose the weight after pregnancy, it is also going to help you look and feel better. Eating omega 3 fatty acids helps reduce inflammation, meaning less pressure on your joints. Eating healthy fats is going to help your body; consuming more protein is going to create a leaner frame. There are many dietary options for you to follow, and there are a number of ideas out there about dieting. But, eating natural foods, and those which are proven as healthy food sources are going to make you feel better, you will find it easier to think during the day, and you are going to look better, when you are consuming the right, healthy foods.

Consume Vitamin D –

Vitamin D has been proven to help fight certain bone diseases and conditions, and help to strengthen the bones and joints. Not only is this going to make it easier for you to walk and do everyday activities, it is also going to help you move around easily. Getting out in to the sun is a great way to get sufficient Vitamin D in the body; not only that, being in the sun is a great way to help enhance your mood, and to help you feel better, especially if you are having a bad day or suffering from some form of anguish in your day.

Create deadlines –

You are quickly going to learn that as a new mother, you have very little time for yourself. But you have to create deadlines and you have to create a schedule, in order for you to be able to get everything that you have to do, done in the day. It can be as simple as checking of the tasks you have to do around the house, or going out with the baby; if you are a working mom, it might be a little more complex. Regardless of how hectic and busy your life is, when you create deadlines and when you give yourself a schedule to follow, you are going to be a far more productive person, and you are going to find that it is much easier to manage your life. When you have a schedule, this is also going to lead to a healthier lifestyle, as it is going to allow you to eliminate stress, and make sure you get everything you have to do done in a day.

Create goals –

If you create goals for yourself to achieve, you will find that you are not only going to feel more productive when you reach one of them, you are also going to find that this simple habit can help you lead a healthier lifestyle. Goals should be set for everything you want to accomplish; whether they are big or small, a goal is a great way for you to see where you were, and where you want to be once you complete that set or specified goal. It does not matter how meaningless or trivial it may seem, when you complete something that you have set out to do, you are going to feel accomplished and you are going to feel a sense of entitlement, which is a great way for you to move forward, and become a better person in life.

Create new experiences –

A great way for you to grow, not only as a mother, but as a person, is to set new experiences and challenges up for yourself. You should always want to try new things, and do things that you never thought you could accomplish. When you set up new experiences, whether it is once a week, once a month, or once a year, you are going to push yourself to try new things that you never thought you were going to be able to do. By doing this, not only are you going to feel accomplished once you do that task, you are also going to learn something new. When we learn, we are continually growing, and we are always improving ourselves; so, it should be something that you would never want or believe you could do, in order to push yourself, and grow along the way as well.

Make a clean home –

No matter how big or small your home is, you should be in an environment that you feel happy in. When things are thrown all over the room or when your home is a mess and cluttered, you are going to find it impossible to think clearly. You should not work in these conditions, and you should not raise your child in these conditions. So, making a clean work area, and keeping your home clean at all times, is a great way to feel stress free, and to feel at ease when you are at home. You want to place yourself in a location you are comfortable in, and when your home is clean and clutter free, you are going to find it is much easier to function, and your mind is also going to work through things far easier, when you do not have to work through clutter.

Save –

We always complain about money, yet we do not look at the little things we do each day, which we could otherwise save. Some of us drink a cup or two of coffee out of the house each day; some buy lunch every day. No matter what you are doing that is costing you more money, there are a number of small things you can do each day, to put a little bit aside. Not only is this going to make it easier for you to be able to supply for your family and child, it is also a great way for you to teach your child (as they get older), how to save. It might be as simple as making coffee at home or bringing lunch with you a couple of days each week. No matter what it is, you will find that there are things you can do, and there are places that you can cut back, to help you save.

Destress –

You stress about everything in life. From work and the family, to financials, and other things you deal with in life. If you are a stressed person, this is going to flow down to your children. You have to find something that is going to help you relax each day. For some people it is going to the gym and getting in an intense workout, for others it is reading a book, and for some it is simply going outside and getting some much-needed sunlight during the day. No matter what it is that helps you calm down, you have to find a few things you can do to help eliminate the stress you feel each day. This is going to help calm you down, and it is going to help you lead a healthier and better life.

It does not matter what kind of life you lead, how much (or little) money you have, what kind of job you work, or what stresses you are dealing with in life, you have to find lifestyle habits that not only help eliminate the stress in your life, but also work to make you a better person. There are many things that you can do, and there are many habits you can create, which are not only going to help improve you and your overall self being, but as a new parent, they are also going to resonate with your child.

You might believe that at such a young age your newborn does not see you struggling or see the stress that you are dealing with, but they can sense it. So, you want to bring them up in a stress-free home, and one where you are giving off a positive attitude and vibe. These are a few habits you can try to create, not only to help you eliminate stress you experience, but also to help you become a better person in general. Everyone is different, but we all go through some kind of stress in our lives. These healthy habits can help eliminate certain stresses, and they can help you feel more at ease with your life, and with the difficulties that you are currently going through in your life, regardless of where they are coming from.

Nutrition Guidelines for New Mothers

As a new mom, you have to consider the foods you are putting in to your body, in order to ensure you are getting sufficient nutrition, but also to ensure you are going to start to notice the weight loss after pregnancy. But, if you choose to breast feed, you not only have to consider the food you are getting, but also what you are going to pass on to your child. Weight loss after a baby might seem impossible, or seem like it is going to take quite some time; but, including breast feeding is a great way for you to notice more weight loss, in less time.

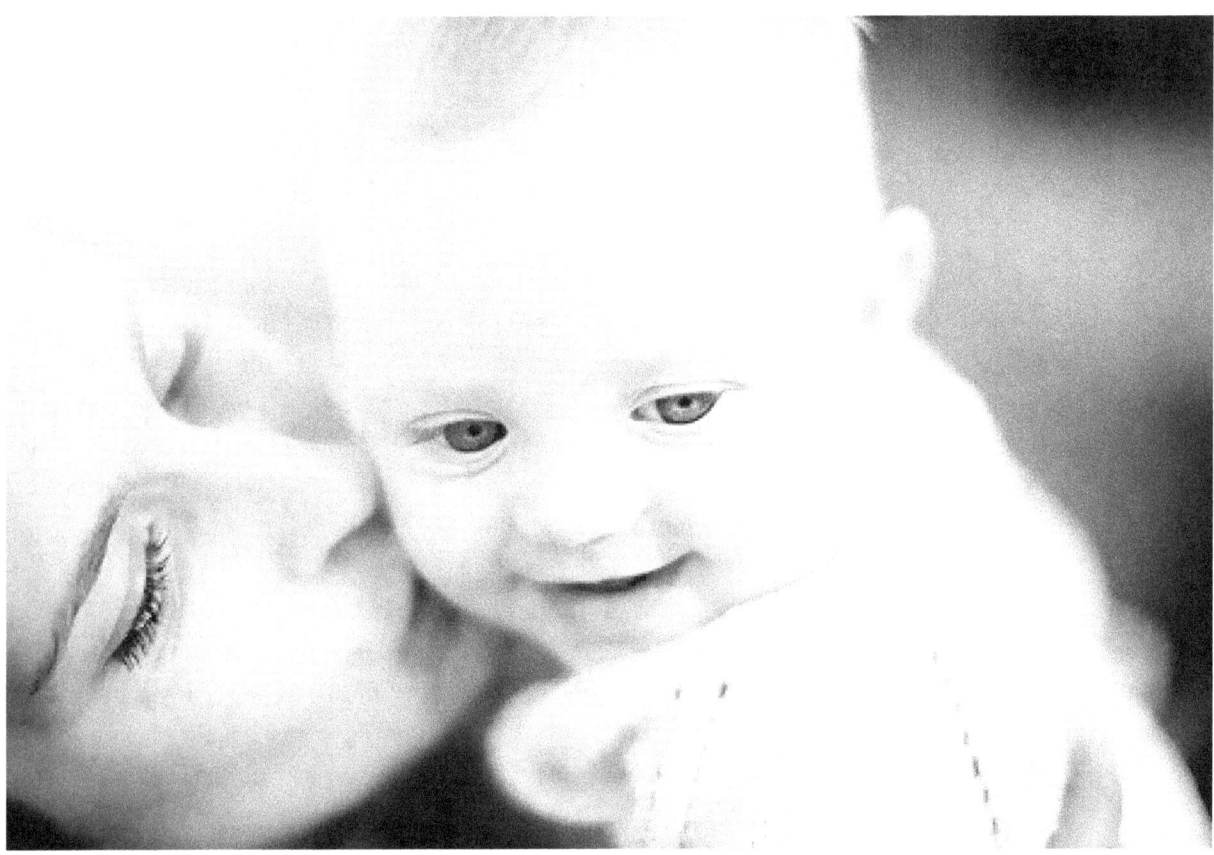

There are certain foods you have to avoid, and certain foods you are going to want to consume. Not only are these healthy for you, but are also going to provide the added nutritious value for your child, when you do choose to breast feed. Regardless of how much you want to lose after pregnancy, the right blend of foods, the right food choices, and eating modified versions of foods you were used to eating while pregnant are all things to consider, in order for you to see the fast weight loss, and still get the necessary nutrients for you and for your baby.

Fish -

Eating fish, namely salmon, is a great way for you to get in your necessary omega 3 fatty acids, and to get high levels of protein. DHA fats are found in high quantities in salmon; this is the fat that is going to provide the "brain" food to your baby if you are breast feeding, and it is beneficial to the joints, and can also help you with memory loss or lapses. Many studies have also shown that it can also help enhance the mood, and help with postpartum depression which many women tend to suffer from after giving birth. Although it is a great food, there are recommendations for women to consider eating no more than 12 oz per week, and this is to limit the amount of mercury that goes in to the milk if you are breastfeeding your child.

Dairy -
If you choose to include dairy, make it low fat. Dairy, whether it is yogurt or a glass of milk, is going to provide you with various essential vitamins including B and D, which you might not be getting through other food sources that are included in the diet. And, if you are breastfeeding, it is going to help with calcium levels, and producing the healthiest milk for your baby, so they are going to receive the highest levels of calcium, and you are going to receive the necessary fat in your diet, through a healthy source after pregnancy.

Lean beef -
Another great food to include in the diet is lean beef, as it is very high in protein which is essential in your diet after pregnancy. Not only is a high protein diet essential for quick weight loss after pregnancy, it is also going to give you the fuel and energy that you need to get through the day, after giving birth and having to take care of a newborn. Vitamin B 12 is also found in high quantities in lean meat sources, so it is a great way for you to get the added protein in to your diet, and it is a good way for you to get in essential vitamins and minerals, even though you are only eating a few ounces of the lean beef or meat during the week.

Legumes -
Iron is also essential to your diet after pregnancy, and it should also be consumed by your child, so legumes are a great source, which are very high in iron levels. And, for those who are vegetarians and are not getting enough protein post pregnancy, consuming legumes is a great way for you to consume more protein, and get in the essential iron levels. Legumes are also a great choice for weight loss after pregnancy, as they are extremely high in fiber; fiber not only fills you up quickly, it is also going to help you consume less during the course of the day, so you are going to notice more weight loss, in a shorter period of time when you are consuming more beans and legumes.

Berries -
Blueberries and strawberries are a great source of antioxidants, not only for you but also for your child. They are also very high in vitamins and minerals that are essential to the body, and they provide you with a healthy option for carbohydrates, without packing on the calories. You can consume them in a shake, you can eat them on their own, or you can add them to a meal; regardless of how you choose to consume them, berries are a great addition to your diet after you have given birth, and they are a great source of antioxidants for both you and for your child.

Oranges -
 You can skip the juice and the pills, when you want high sources of calcium and vitamin C, oranges are quite possibly the best option for you to turn to. Citrus is also excellent when you are breastfeeding, and they provide you with more energy as a new mom, which is something that every new mother need. Additionally, oranges make a great snack, they are easy to carry around with you anywhere, and they are a great source of energy if you are feeling tired, and need something to eat, but do not want to consume a calorie heavy meal. And, if you consume an orange prior to your meal, you are going to find that you will limit the number of calories that you are going to consume during any meal, which is a simple solution to help you consume fewer calories each day, and help you notice faster weight loss after you have just given birth.

Brown rice -
 Although you think cutting back on carbs is a must for weight loss, you can't cut back too much if you are breastfeeding, as this will reduce the amount of milk that you produce. So, when you do choose carbs, make sure to choose a healthy source like brown rice; it helps produce the essential calories that your body needs to produce more milk, you only have to consume limited quantities in order to reach those levels, and this food is extremely high in fiber, which is going to help keep you regular, and help fill you up faster, so you are not going to consume as much when you eat brown rice with a meal or other source of protein.

Eggs -
 Like salmon, eggs have high levels of DHA which is essential for you and your baby; additionally, eggs provide you with a great source of protein, and they are going to provide you with a good healthy fat. If you choose to eat eggs, only consume one yolk (if you consume 3 eggs, eat one yolk, and three egg whites). Egg whites are extremely low in calories, and are going to provide you with a very high source of protein. They are also a great source to snack on, as you can boil them, and keep them in the refrigerator for a snack if you find that you get hungry, but do not want to consume a larger meal, you can simply eat a couple of eggs to fill you up during the day.

Wheat -
 If you do consume bread, cereal, and other wheat, go with whole wheat. It provides high sources of folic acid, which is crucial to your child's development during the earlier years of life. When they are fortified, these sources of fuel are also going to provide you with a variety of healthy and necessary vitamins and minerals that the body needs. Whether it is whole wheat pasta, or a couple slices of toast, you want to go with the darker, whole wheat options, when you choose to consume these foods. And, like other high fiber foods, when you choose whole wheat, you are getting a higher source of fiber per serving, meaning you are likely going to consume less during the meals, and you are going to eat less during the course of the day, both which are going to bode well for weight loss after pregnancy.

Leafy greens -
Vitamin A is also a source that is essential to your child's development, and is needed by the mother, if

they are breast feeding. Food sources like spinach or lettuce, broccoli and other leafy greens are going to provide this. They are also extremely low in calories, and make a great meal source, and work as a binder, if you are going to include them with a high protein source for your meals during the day. Veggies which are green are also very high in antioxidant levels, which are going to help enhance your mood and are needed for both mom and baby, especially if the mother is breastfeeding her child.

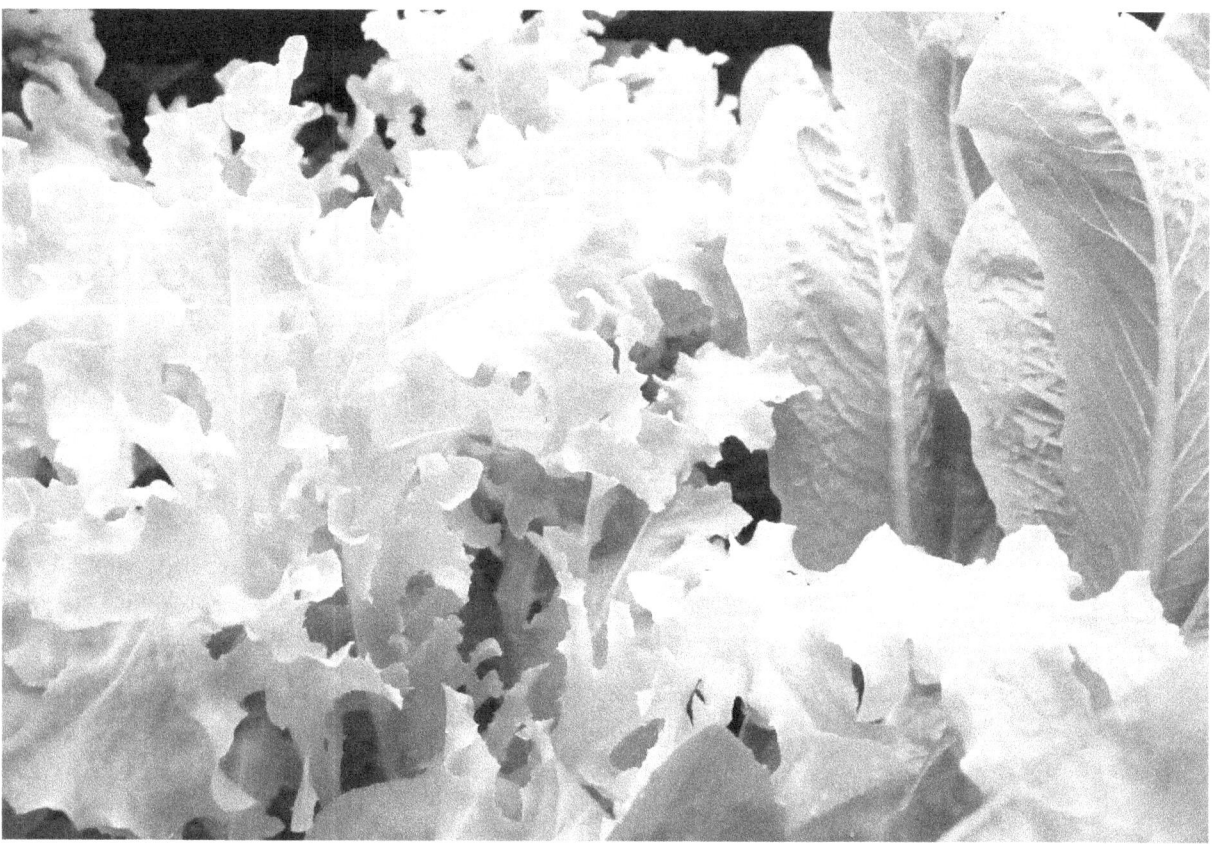

Nuts -

 A great snack food are nuts; whether you choose almonds, walnuts, or any other source, they are a great food to consume. They are very high in healthy fats, they are going to provide you a source of fiber, and nuts are great to help you fight off hunger. If you notice you are hungry during the day, consuming a handful of nuts is a great way for you to keep away the hunger, and to consume less, the next time you do consume a meal. Nuts are also high in vitamins, and produce essential fats to the mother and baby, which are needed for development, and for healthy diet.

Water -

 In order to ensure you are not dehydrated and your baby is not dehydrated, you have to consume plenty of water. You will also find this helps to flush out your system and helps eliminate any toxins, which is essential if you are breastfeeding, as it is going to ensure your baby is only getting the best and highest sources of fuel in the milk you are feeding it. Additionally, water is necessary to keep the skin looking young and healthy, to help keep you regular, and it is a great way to fill you up. By drinking a large glass of water prior to a meal, and letting it sit in the stomach for a few minutes, you will find that you are going to consume only a fraction of the amount of food you would consume if you did not drink the glass of water prior to eating.

Healthy snacks -
There are many companies that now produce 100 calorie packs, and other similar handy snacks you can take around with you anywhere. These, or a handful of nuts, or a fruit, are all great options to have with you anywhere. If you find you get hungry during the day, this is going to work as a block, to help fill you up until your next meal, and it is also a great way to avoid making the wrong decision, and purchasing a candy bar or other foods you should not be consuming, especially if you are trying to lose weight, and are breastfeeding.

Healthy oils -
When you choose to use oil, use the healthy options. Extra virgin is always the best, and coconut oil is also a great option, as it has been found to help you burn more, and lose more weight, than other sources of oil. You need to get fat in your diet each day, and your baby needs fat; when you use oil, these are the healthy fat sources you should be consuming, and they are the healthy fat choices that you should be giving to your child as well.

Don't count calories -
Post pregnancy, it is not so much about counting calories to lose weight, and if you are breastfeeding, it is something that you really have to avoid. You must remember that you are eating for two; and, when you breastfeed, you are going to burn a few hundred calories a day, so this is going to make up for the additional calories that you are consuming during the course of the day. It is not about counting calories, but instead focusing on what you are consuming, when you are consuming it, and the sources you are choosing for fuel. You have to eat more, as you are feeding two people; but, it is far more important to choose the right sources of fuel, in order to see the best results, to give your baby what they need, and to give your body the fuel it needs, to keep up with the demands that it is going through.

You are naturally going to lose the weight after giving birth; you do not want to focus so much on a calorie restricted diet, but instead going natural, and making the right food choices. When possible, you should go after all natural foods, avoid processed foods as much as possible, and choose the healthier foods which are going to fill you up, and give you the sources of fuel that your body needs, rather than the foods that are going to fill you up for a few minutes, and cause you to feel an empty pit in your stomach about an hour later.

It is not about how little you eat, but the quality of the foods that you are eating after giving birth. These are some of the many foods you are going to want to include in your diet. Not only are they healthy for you, they are also going to give your baby the necessary vitamins and minerals that they need, in order to ensure a healthy and proper development for your child.

How to crush a weight-loss plateau?

Now you know what is plateau and how does it come into being but what you might want to know most of all is how to get rid of it. But just before we go there, it is important to look at your goal. If you have already attained the desired weight and are not willing to lose any more weight than plateau is where you have to stay, but if you want to go further then following are some points that will help you crush that annoying weight-loss plateau.

Make sure you are on a nutritional plan. Your first and foremost step should be to see if you are following a good balanced nutritional plan. You are to make sure that your meal plan fulfills your micro and macro nutrients needs along with proper supply of fiber and water. If you are not on a good plan it will be no use trying to make any changes.

Make sure you are following that meal plan. When you have a meal plan in your hand it is important that you follow it. Because it does not matter how good your plan is it means nothing if you have not been following it religiously. You may have a highly efficient meal plan, but if not followed, it is just a piece of paper. It is important that you reassess you're eating habit and exercise routine. Make sure that you are not taking calories in larger proportions than you should or you are skipping out on your workouts. There is a very important point to consider. You have to be very honest to yourself and with your training program. Let's say you have a goal of consuming 1400 calories a day and you're not weighing out your portions or picking on foods you shouldn't be in between meals that 1400 calories per day will turn into 1700 or even 1900. If your goal is 1400 you need to hit that 1400 no matter what. Yes, it will be a pain in the butt to track and log you're eating in but the only way to achieve permanent fat loss is to change your lifestyle. That means learning how to portion out your food and consuming the right amount of each macronutrient.

Slowly start lowering calories. Now that you are sure that you are following a good nutrition plan you can reduce your calorie intake. The key thing here is do not go overboard with lowering your calories. Don't jump from 1400 calories to 1000 calories. Small little frequent changes will help keep you sane and help you maintain more of your metabolism. I recommend dropping your calories by 50-200 calories every 2-3 weeks depending on your progress.

Increase your cardio. You want to be able to get away with doing as little cardio as possible when trying to drop fat for this reason alone. If you hit a plateau you can slowly increase your cardio 50-100 calories per week. Sometimes all your body needs are a little nudge to get it moving in the right direction.

Be more active. It's not just gym where you can increase your calorie burning. You can do so even in day to day activities. Try walking next time instead of taking car. You can start gardening it will help you physically as well as aesthetically. These small changes in your daily activities can make a lot of difference.

When to make changes to your program

You may have to make changes to your program but before you do make sure that you are following your plan to the T. If you are not you cannot make a change. Dropping calories or increasing your activity will not work if you can't adhere to the program.

You should be monitoring your progress every week. On a weekly basis you should be weighing yourself, taking Bodyfat and measurements. If after 3 weeks with make no progress you can make a minor change, either remove some calories (30-200 calories) or add some cardio work (+100calories of cardio burned). You need to keep track of every change your body makes during this time. Once you make a change you need to monitor progress, if the scale isn't moving still wait another 3 weeks. Our bodies do not want to be lean; being lean is hard for our bodies to manage. The human body wants to carry around extra fat, fat does nothing but insult. Fat loss is not a quick linear process; you are going to have ups and downs. There will be weeks when the fat seems to be flying off while other weeks when you feel stuck. Either way it will take some time to drop fat. Healthy weight loss is .5-2lbs per week, when you lose more weight than that you risk the chance of your body losing muscle and slowing down your metabolism.

Eat Healthier Than Ever Before!

If you want to lose the weight after a child or keep from gaining too much, eating healthier is more important than ever. Yes, even during pregnancy, and that isn't easy to do. Eating healthy is more than just avoiding cravings during and after pregnancy, but what you eat really will affect your weight immensely. This chapter will take you through eating healthy while pregnant to losing weight by eating healthy. There are tips and tricks that will help you along the way too.

Why Eat Healthy While Pregnant:

Even if you are eating more than just what you would normally if you didn't have a child, you don't need to be eating unhealthily. It's not good for you or for the developing baby. You both need the proper nutrition if you want to be healthy during the pregnancy and to deliver a healthy child. Remember that during t4he first trimester, you probably don't need to add anything to your diet, but just stay healthy and in shape so that you can provide the best for the developing fetus. In the second trimester, you can eat healthy but that doesn't mean to eat a lot.

You'll notice that you are less hungry and experience less cravings when you are getting enough nutrition. Remember that just because you're eating healthy while pregnant this does not mean that you are dieting while you are pregnant. You want to make slow lifestyle changes that will be better for you and the baby. Don't just cut out food and try to lose weight. You're simply trying to avoid putting on more weight than needed so it's less weigh to lose later.

Tips to Eat Healthy While Pregnant:

Here are some tips and tricks to help you eat healthy while pregnant without risking going into dieting territory. This will keep you from gaining the excess pounds that you'll have to lose later on.

- Throw Away the Junk: The first and easiest thing to do is to throw away the junk food. You'll eat healthier food if that's the options you have. You won't want to wait, and this will avoid the temptation of bad habits that you're sure to regret later.

- Eat Breakfast: It's easy to forget breakfast at any normal time. No less when you're pregnant. During pregnancy mornings can be rough. You may have morning sickness or at the very least an upset stomach. Try whole wheat toast, saving food for later in the morning but kick starting your metabolism so you don't gain those extra pounds. Fortified cereals will also help because they're easy as well as having extra nutrients.

- Eat Food with Fiber: Fiber is your best friend when trying not to gain excess weight when pregnant, and there are many fruits and vegetables that have it. For example, try cooked greens, melon, bananas and even carrots. Beans and whole grains, such as rice and oatmeal will also help. This will keep your digestive tract running smoothly as well as your metabolism. It also keeps you full longer.

- Healthy Snacks: You want to have healthy snacks on hand if you don't want to choose an unhealthy option or eat too many large meals. Low fat or fat free yogurt is great, especially with fresh fruit. If you're craving dairy, try low-fat cheese or whole grain crackers if you just want to munch on something.

- No Soft Cheese or Lunch Meat: This is something that most people don't think about, but they actually have bacteria that may harm your child. For example, stay away from brie, goat cheeses or cheeses like feta. Lunch meats and hotdogs may be bad for the baby as well unless they are heated until they are steaming hot. It has the same effect as undercooked meat like sushi.

- Limit Caffeine: This goes all the way back to hydration. Caffeine will dehydrate you, and it can hurt you and the child.

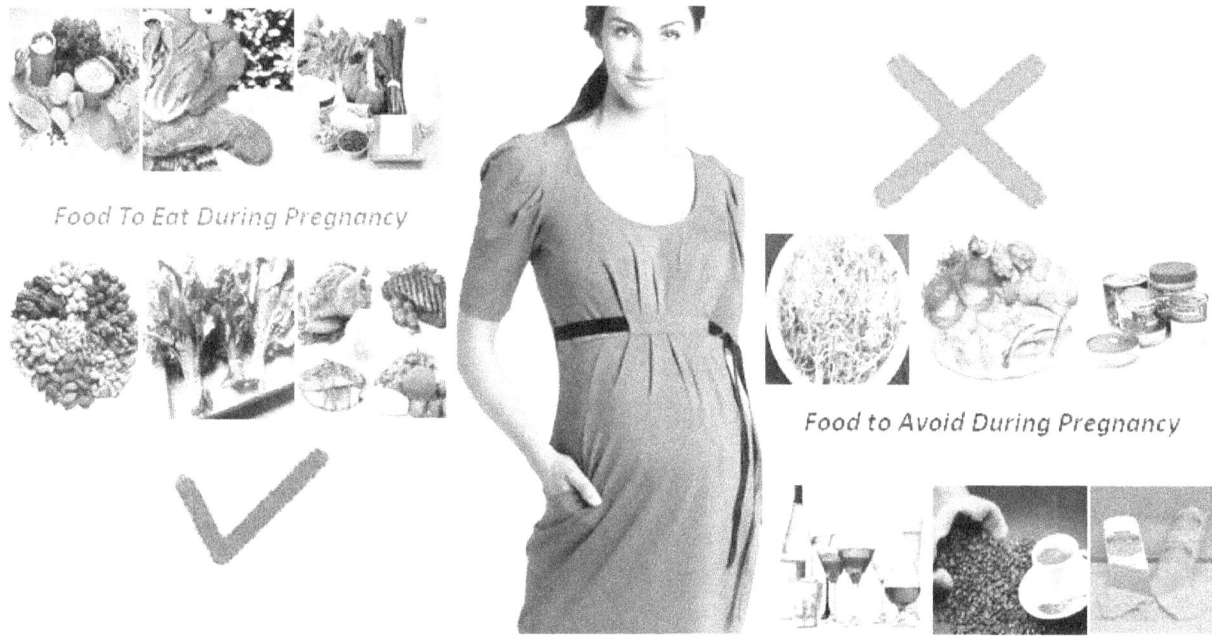

Food To Eat During Pregnancy

Food to Avoid During Pregnancy

Why Healthy Eating Affects Weight Loss:

What you eat will obviously determine your weight. If you did give into those cravings or gained too much weight despite your efforts, you can still lose weight after you've given birth. If you're eating nothing but fatty foods, then you can't be surprised when your body stores fat. There are some foods that are easier to burn than others as well. For example, it is easier for you to burn rice, especially brown rice, versus pasta. You need to know what to eat to lose weight. With just exercise, you will lose some weight, but you can be severely hindered by not having the proper diet.

More Tips to Help You Eat Healthy & Lose Weight:

Here are some tips that will help you eat to lose weight with a daily exercise regime. These tricks will make eating healthy a little easier of a feat to accomplish.

- Portion Size Matters: Portion size is extremely important when you're trying to accomplish healthy eating. Many people find that eating four to six times a day in smaller portions will keep you from unhealthy snacking or eating too much at once. It can even keep you from indulging too much in something that is bad for you.

- Time Your Time: You need to take your time when eating or your body won't register when it's full. This can cause cramping as well.

- Avoid Sugary Drinks: You need to avoid sugary drinks when you're trying to lose weight an exercise. They will make you feel sluggish, slow your metabolism down, and they have empty calories.

- Slowly Make Changes: You can't just change everything at once and expect it to stick. When you're adding in dietary changes and exercise routines, you can't expect to stick to a drastic overhaul. You need to make small changes that will go a long way, such as exercising for fifteen to thirty minutes a day and cutting down to one soda a day.

- More Fiber: Again, always keep more fiber in your diet. It's good for your digestive track, and it stays in your stomach longer, meaning you'll eat less overall.

- Don't Snack: You're going to snack occasionally, and when you do you need to make sure that you're choosing healthy snacks. Of course, try to avoid snacking entirely or at least regulate the snacks to make sure you know exactly how many calories you're going to be consuming that day.

- Leafy Greens: Leafy greens will aid in weight loss, and it increases the volume of your meals without adding extra calories that aren't needed. They are also a great source of vitamins, antioxidants and minerals. It can even add calcium into your diet, and they can help to aid in fat burning.

- Lean Meats: Lean meats are good for you, and meat shouldn't be demonized. It's good for you, and you can eat beef if it's lean beef. Protein is a fulfilling nutrient, and eating a high protein diet can help you to burn eighty to a hundred more calories each and every day. It can even cut your cravings down, allowing you to lose more pounds each and every week.

- Soups are a Must: Low energy density is a good way to eat because it contains lots of water, fruits, and vegetables, and this will help you to hydrate as well.

- Nuts: This is a great, healthy snack to add in to your diet, but it is high in fat. That does not necessarily mean that it is satisfying.

Workouts for While the Baby Naps

With a newborn in the house, it can be difficult to find time to do anything at all for yourself. Finding time to exercise can be almost impossible, especially if you're a single mother or your partner isn't around for whatever reason. However, there are still workout routines that you can use to help you lose the baby weight. Each of the workouts in this section are ten-minute exercises that you can fit in anytime the baby naps. When a newborn nap, they'll usually be out for at least ten minutes. Fit in more exercise whenever you can, but if ten minutes at a time is all you have, then you should take full advantage of it if you want to get back to your pre-baby body.

Try Out Lotta Tabata:

This is a great way to increase your heart rate in a short period of time, but you probably shouldn't do it until you ask your doctor if it's okay, especially if you had a C-section. You'll do twenty seconds of hard, intense workout, and then you'll follow each twenty second sprint with ten seconds of rest. When doing a Tabata, you'll do eight intervals total so that you get to four full minutes. Work at your own pace and at your own level, and make sure that you always take breaks as needed. This is an advanced form of exercise, and it can be adapted to you no matter what fitness level you're on. You can try pushups, burpees, plank or squats depending on what you feel most comfortable with. Change it up each session, but make sure that you do the same thing for each of the eight intervals in one session.

A Little Cardio Blasting:

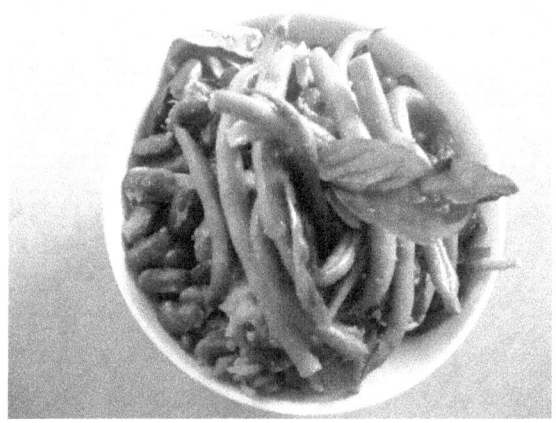

This is a workout where you will complete a full minute of intense cardio and then you'll move onto the next exercise. This will work as a type of circuit, doing one exercise after another. This will get your heart pumping, and it'll keep it elevated for the ten to twenty minutes that you have to maximize the calorie burning that you do while your child naps. Start with butt kicks, jump rope, ret, mountain climbers, and so forth. You can even add jogging in place and jumping jacks depending on what you feel you're up to and what your doctor approves.

Full Body Routine:

This is a great way to incorporate weight training, which will help you to shed the pounds from excessively stubborn areas. You'll only need dumbbells for this exercise, and you don't even need them to be heavy. Make sure that you repeat the series two to three times, and with each exercise you'll want to do ten to twelve reps.

- Start with a minute of jumping jacks or jump rope.

- Go to triceps kickbacks next.

- Move forward with bicep curls.

- Then you'll want to go to your basic pushups.

- Do dumbbell rows next, and then move on to lunges.

- You can then do squats, and then do a minute in plank.

Belly Slim Workout:

One of the areas that needs the most attention after having a child is usually the stomach, and this exercise helps you to target the abs that you lost. You'll want to repeat the following series at least two to three times if possible, and make sure that every exercise on the list is performed for at least a fully sixty seconds.

- Start with a traditional crunch.

- Move on to a bicycle crunch.

- Then a reverse crunch.

- A feet up crunch is next.

- Then go back to plank.

Some Positions Explained:

There are some positions in this section that you may not know what are, and that can make it almost impossible for you to be able to do the exercises above to lose the weight that you no longer need or want. This section is dedicated to making sure that you know how to do each position in proper form which will shed the pounds and help you to avoid injury. Never try to perform a position that you don't understand, and always ask your doctor before you start any new exercise routine to avoid injury after having a child.

- Burpees: Begin by standing, and then you'll lower your body into a squatting position. While you do this, you'll want to keep your hands on the floor. They should be placed in front of you, and then kick your feet backwards, lowering down into a pushup. Lower yourself until your chest touches the floor, pushing back up and resuming the squatting position afterward. Then, perform a vertical jump as high as you can before repeating.

- Bicep Curls: To do bicep curls, you'll start by holding a dumbbell in each hand. Make sure you're standing with your feet a hip distance apart again. Curl both of your arms upward, but make sure the dumbbells stay in line with your shoulders. Your abs should be tight with your knees slightly bent.

- Mountain Climber: A mountain climber will have you starting in plank position, with your weight resting on the balls of your feet. Then you'll bring a leg forward to your chest, moving it back to starting position afterwards. Alternate legs, and always remember to keep breathing.

- Butt Kicks: Butt kicks are helpful when trying to lose weight too, but they do no good if you don't know the proper form to do them in. you'll need to stand, and your feet should face forward but also be hip distance apart from each other. You'll then contract your glutes, bringing your right heel up to your glutes, and then allow the foot to land, and repeat with the other side. Make sure you do not arch your back while doing a butt kick.

- Triceps Kickbacks: You'll start by leaning forward, and you'll do this from your hips until you're at about a forty-five-degree angle to the floor. Your back should stay straight, but bend your elbows until your upper arms are made parallel to the floor. Your upper arms need to stay still, but straight your arm behind your body, making sure that your back stays flat and your elbows stay close to your waist.

- Planks: When you're doing a high plank, you should make sure that your hands are directly under your shoulders, and your arms should remain straight. Your legs need to be straight back, and this will keep your tailbone tucked as well as your abs tight. Then, you'll lower yourself down. This is a basic pushup position, and when you're trying to add difficulty you can do a forearm plank. This is where you lower your forearms to the ground with your palms facing down, and your elbow should be directly under your shoulders.

- Lunges: Keep your feet at hips distance apart, and then take a large step forward with your right leg, lower your hips down until your legs are at a ninth-degree angle, and then repeat.

- Reverse Crunches: We've already covered traditional crunches, but reverse crunches are essential to helping lose that stubborn belly fat as well. Your feet need to be flat on the ground when you start, bending your legs at the knee, raising your feet so that your knees are now over your hips. Make sure that your abs are contracted, and lift your knee towards your chest and then lower back and hips should be off the ground. Alternate.

- Bicycle Crunches: Lay flat on the floor, and lift your knees to a forty-five-degree angle. Your elbow should touch to the opposite knee, twisting back and forth. This mimic riding a bike.

- Feet up Crunches: This is the same movement as when you start a traditional crunch, but your legs will be extended straight up instead of having your feet flat to the floor. Keep your feet where they're in line with your hips, and contract your abs. lift your head and torso off the floor.

- Dumbbell Rows: Your knees need to stay bent, leaning forward form your hips. Let your arms hang down but also a bit forward. Your arms will then be pulled up until your elbow is pointing at the ceiling, and your upper arm should be parallel to the floor. Keep the back straight and brace your abs for the exercise.

Returning to Exercise

Everyone's journey back to exercise will be different physically and mentally. Show yourself and another moms grace during this period. Each new mom will heal at different rates, and although it's important for your body to heal the first few weeks, no judgment should be cast on one another for how quickly or slowly one returns to fitness. Hopefully, the education in the previous chapter highlights the importance of why it's key to be intentional in your healing postpartum. And then it's up to you to know your own body and mind and what your limitations and modifications will be. Ask for help if you're not sure.

Your return to exercise will vary greatly based upon

- your previous exercise levels.

- any complications during pregnancy, labor, and birth (including tearing, stitches, cesarean, intensity of labor, trauma).

- how well your pelvic floor and abdominal muscles are healing or working.

- mental state: some may experience a tough time holding themselves back from pushing too hard, and others may have a hard time motivating themselves to get moving in a meaningful way.

Whatever your fitness goals may be now, it's important to have a plan. If you've ever watched someone recover from a major trauma, surgery, or bed rest, there's often a guided rehab protocol that one would move through slowly and steadily. As your initial exercises get easier, then continue to advance them. Being postpartum, you have a new normal, and therefore it's great to have an actual game plan. Maybe even write it out. I'll go through a few examples of returning to cardio and strength training. Modify the suggestions to fit your interests and level of fitness.

Connect with your breath

Your diaphragm, the breathing muscle along the bottom of the ribs and the muscle that represents the roof of the core, most likely became tightened and constricted while baby was growing. Now is your chance to make sure you can find a nice, full breath again. Take a breath in, and you should feel not only your chest and belly expand, but also your ribs to the sides and in the back. When you exhale and let the air out, those areas should sink back down. Inhale = expand in all directions; exhale = relax, sink back down.

As you move your body from a sitting position to standing, while you lift your baby, or while you reach for something, practice exhaling (blowing the air out of your mouth) during the exertion. Take a full breath in and then exhale and move. This is an easy way to optimize the pressure inside your body and start getting your core muscles, pelvic floor, and lower abdomen to coordinate again. Some cues that might help you remember to do this without making it a forceful exhalation and to avoid gripping your abdominals would be to pretend you are cooling soup on a spoon or blowing out through a straw when you move.

Posture

Your posture may have changed while you were pregnant to accommodate your growing baby, but now that baby is out and being carried around, you may notice that you still fall back into pregnancy posture. Changing up your posture itself is an exercise. Try to find a relatively neutral pelvic position most of the

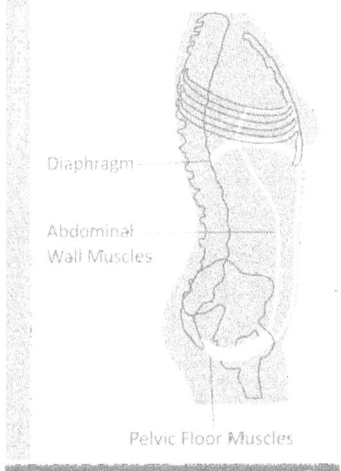

Diaphragm

Abdominal
Wall Muscles

Pelvic Floor Muscles

juliewiebept.com

time, meaning you don't want to tuck your tailbone/butt under and have a flat back, but you also don't want to untuck to the extreme and arch your back to the max. Go between those two directions a few times, and then try to find the middle ground. Most new moms tend to live with their butt tucked under, so try to untuck and use those glutes (your butt muscles)! Now that your pelvis can move more easily, try to align your ribs over your pelvis. This will optimize your body's pressure system inside the core (diaphragm on top, pelvic floor on the bottom). Ribs over pelvis means not leaning so far back that your ribs are flared forward and not so rounded forward in your chest and shoulders that there's no room in the core.

The concept of a pressure relationship between the diaphragm and the pelvic floor (and much more!) is taught as Piston Science created and owned by Julie Wiebe, PT. For over 20 years, she has been integrating these concepts and strategies into movement, function, and all forms of fitness, including running, CrossFit and more. Julie has also been an advocate for empowering women to pursue fitness in the midst of pelvic health and pain issues. She is internationally recognized for pioneering the integrative approach that is now widely relied upon by physical therapists and fitness professionals, including me. Her information is used with permission. For more information about Julie, please visit her website, blogs, videos, and online courses. Links are located in the Resources appendix.

Pelvic floor

Your pelvic floor muscles are those that connect from the pubic bone in the front to the tailbone in the back and your sit bones side to side. They are internal muscles that wrap around all three openings (urethra, vagina, anus) and attach to various depths in that region. It is a group of muscles that work together to keep your organs up and inside of you, to keep you from leaking, and to provide support and stability.

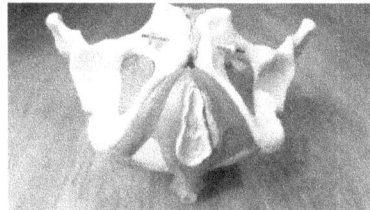 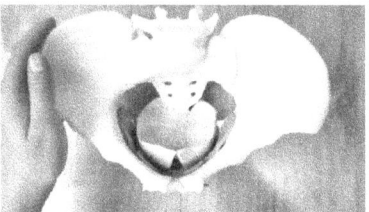

To begin connecting with your pelvic floor, find the diaphragm breath we just talked about, and add a relaxation of the pelvic floor with your inhale and a contraction of the pelvic floor with your exhale. It's also important to sometimes practice lengthening your pelvic floor on an exhale to help you relax when urinating or having a bowel movement. To focus on the relax portion, visualize your pelvic floor letting go, melting like butter, opening like a flower. To focus on the contraction portion, visualize yourself closing your vaginal opening around a kidney bean and lifting the bean up and into your body, stopping from peeing, stopping from passing gas, pulling the pubic bone and tailbone up and into your body, and pulling the sit bones up and into your body.

- Inhale = relax pelvic floor = let kidney bean go.

- Exhale = contract pelvic floor = lift the kidney bean up and in.

Repeat.

Putting it together

As we start to plan out our return to exercise, please keep this strategy in mind. In any exercise you try — walking, lifting, running, rowing, jumping — you should be able to feel yourself find a full breath and that your pelvic floor can follow your breath and contract and relax as you need it to.

Add this strategy to simple movements with only five to ten repetitions with a focus on quality.

The strategy of inhale + relax, then exhale + contract + move can be applied to following real life activities, as exercises, before you begin your full return to exercise:

Sit to stand from a chair

Lifting baby

Picking up an object from the ground

Lifting your stroller in and out of the car

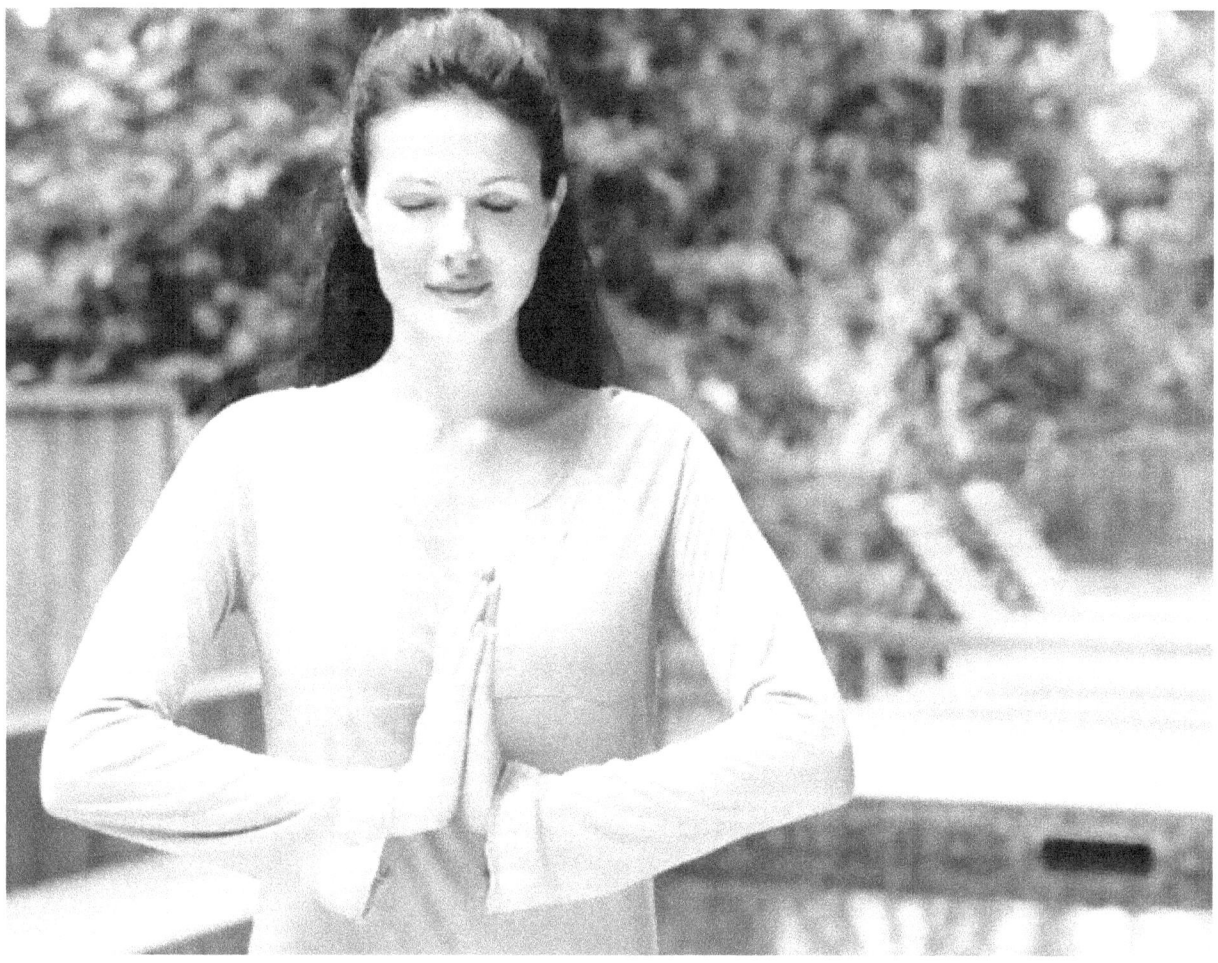

Return to Cardio

The ways you can vary your progression include: distance, total time, speed, and predictable versus variable terrain/conditions.

Example for returning to walking, jogging, running, hiking

Start with small frequent walks: five minutes in length at a slow to normal speed. After a few days like this with no feelings of pain, leakage or falling out, start to increase time or distance.

Progress walks to be ten to fifteen minutes at your normal speed.

Continue to lengthen the time of your walks in five- to ten-minute increments at your normal speed.

Advance the total time of your walks or start to vary speed in intervals. If your end goal is jogging or running, you can start to add in very small intervals of jogging a block or 30 seconds to a minute, then return to walking for a few minutes before once again jogging for a short period of time. You should continue checking in with your body during and after these advancements to monitor for pain, leakage, or pelvic heaviness.

Continue to change up lengthening the speed portions of jog/run with walking to slowly build up to more jogging/running than walking.

Vary terrain to trails, hills, and uneven surfaces as you feel stronger.

The example above could take some new moms' weeks or months or years. It really depends so much on how your body is responding. This is different from one woman to the next and from one pregnancy to the next. Leaking or feeling like something is falling out is not something to push through. You may find that you can increase your time just fine, but once you add in speed, you start to leak. Or maybe it's not the change of speed, but at a certain distance or on hills you notice symptoms. Stop and modify. Keep staying active, but don't push into the symptoms. If they aren't resolving on their own or with your intentional pelvic floor exercises, breath, and posture, reach out to a professional specializing in postpartum recovery (links in Resources appendix) to get an assessment and develop a plan specific to your needs.

Return to Strength

The ways you can vary your progression include: weights, body position, repetitions, sets, total time, and intensity or speed.

Example for squats

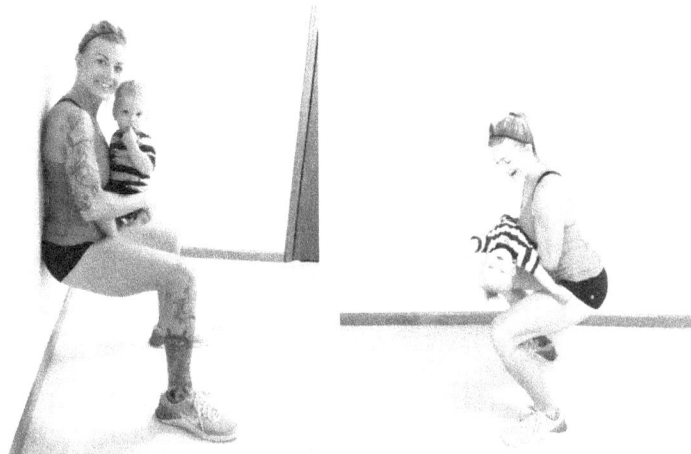

Start with holding on to a countertop, railing, sturdy chair, or with your back against a wall. Work on getting your form, breath, and pelvic floor coordinated with the movement. Perform a maximum of ten repetitions at one time so you can focus on quality. Slowly increase repetitions by five or by the number of times you're performing the squats per day.

Advance by performing squats without weight yet, but no holding on anymore. Perform to a depth you feel comfortable with and continue to focus on form, breath, and pelvic floor. Continue to perform only ten repetitions. Increase repetitions over time by five or by number of times you're performing per day.

Start to add weights to your squats. Hold your baby or pick something less than 20 pounds to start with. Perform squats with the weight or baby around chest height. Continue to add reps/sets as it gets easier. Continue to have a strong focus on quality and no pain, leakage, or feelings of falling out.

If that's your goal, continue to increase weights — barbell, kettlebell, water jugs, baby, etc. — in different positions, keeping the weight light and getting used to different lifts again. Ensure quality and connection to pelvic floor with no symptoms.

Ease back into whatever your new squat goals are — depth, reps, weight, speed, etc. Continue to listen to your body. Vary challenges by performing single leg squats or adding a rotational component.

Again, the example above may take some women weeks, months, or years to progress through, based on their own unique circumstances.

Example for push-ups

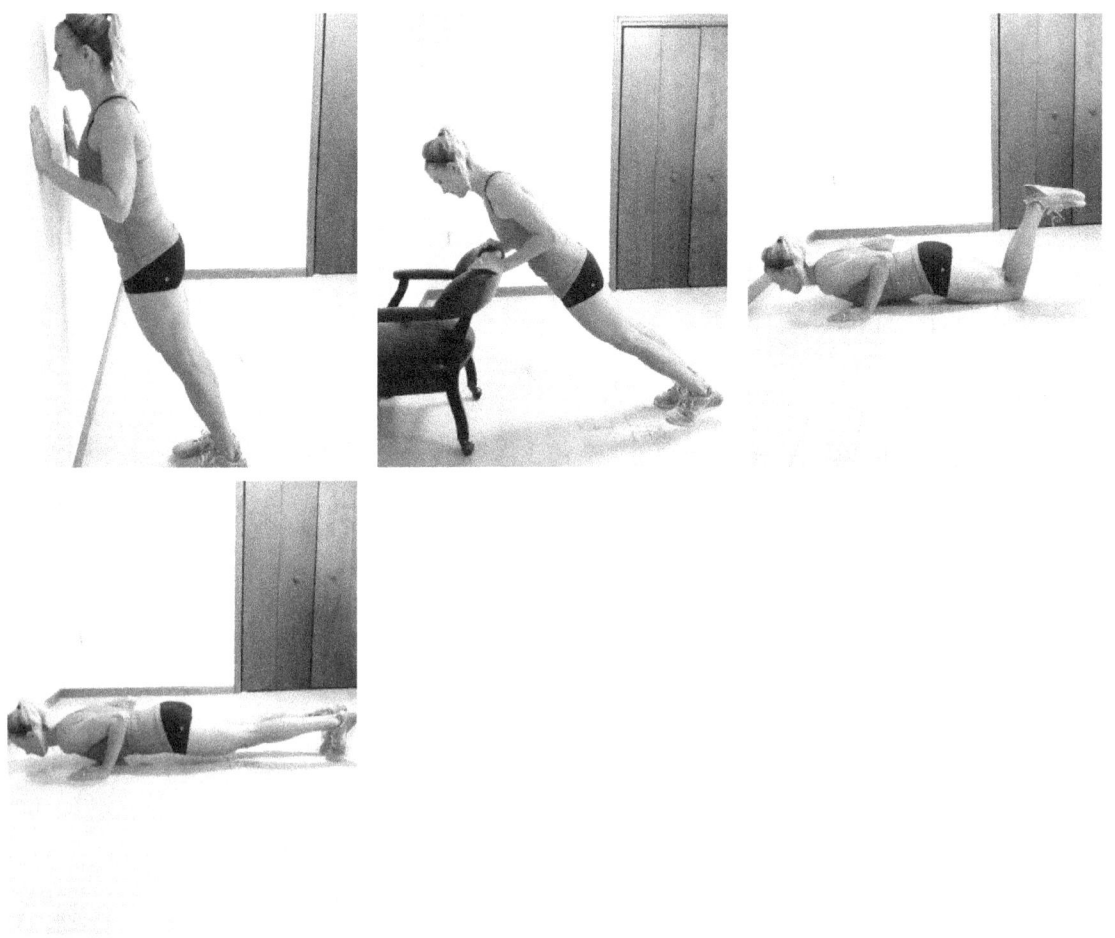

Start doing push-ups against a wall or countertop and focus on breath and pelvic floor coordination.

Continue to increase repetitions at the previous height or decrease distance to floor.

Progress to floor push-ups from knees or plank position. Keep reps low at five to ten as you focus on form, breath, and pelvic floor.

Continue to increase total reps/sets or challenge yourself with different placements of your hands.

Example for plank progression

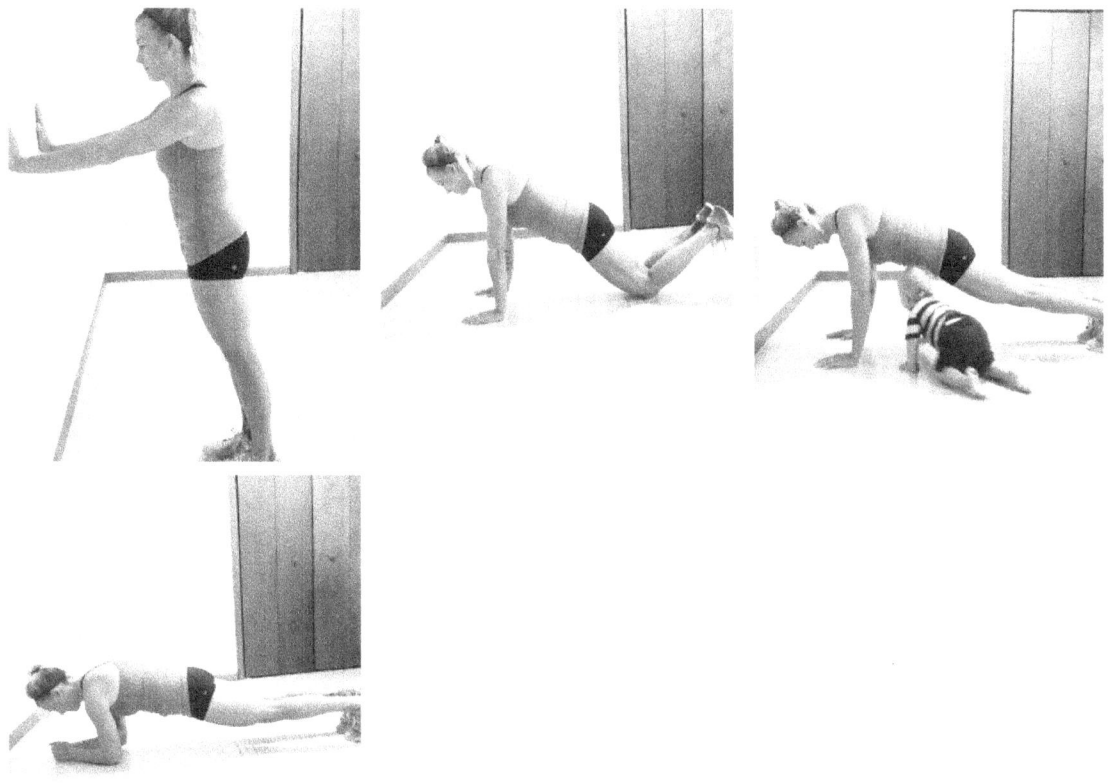

Start in a modified position similar to push-up positions: on the wall, countertop, or couch if needed. Time the length of your plank holds with just one or two breath cycles to begin rather than counting total time in the plank position. Breath cycle: inhale and exhale gently (don't hold your breath).

Increase number of breath cycles in those positions, and then slowly make your way to the floor. Plank from knees. Plank using straight arms. Plank using forearms. Monitor for symptoms and doming/coning of the abdomen, and continue to connect with pelvic floor, breath, and posture.

As you're able to hold the plank position longer, add in more functional challenges. You could add movement of arms with shoulder taps, reaching out, or alternate between forearm and hands during the hold. Or you could add movement of the legs with leg lifts up or tap a leg to the side.

Return to jumping

Just because you had a baby does not mean you're doomed to exile from the trampoline for fear of peeing your pants, nor does it mean that you should perform jumping jacks and double under (jump roping where you pass the rope through twice in one jump) as much as you want and ignore or embrace the leakage. You do not have to live with leakage, and if you want to be able to jump dry, you should!

Start with squatting, and as you come up from the squat, extend up onto your toes to mimic getting ready for a jump. Practice your breathing and pelvic floor coordination with this modification.

Practice one small jump with exhale and with a pelvic floor contraction during the takeoff and landing.

Slowly increase the height of the jump or the number of jumps in a row. For example, breathe in, then exhale/jump twice, then inhale-relax-break, then exhale/jump twice, then rest. Slowly increase the number of jumps in a row or height of the jump very intentionally so that you can notice specifically where/if you have any symptoms occur. Is it just on higher jumps, is it the takeoff versus the landing, or is it just past rep eight?

If you know when symptoms are occurring, you'll be able to better modify and not push past the limitations of what your body is capable of. If you're having trouble getting back into this, work with a pelvic floor PT or postnatal fitness specialist, who can help you with a more thorough assessment of what you have going on and the coordination and timing.

Hopefully, you're able to use the above progressions to modify to the exercises you enjoy doing and come up with a plan of how to ease back into your movements intentionally. If you are experiencing any pain, leakage, pelvic heaviness, or coning/doming, reach out for help. It does not necessarily mean your muscles are weak! There's a lot at play including your connective tissues' role in healing. Difficulty with the coordination may include: ability to contract and relax your pelvic floor and abdominal muscles, tight muscles or scar tissue, and injury/trauma sustained during labor/birth. Lots of times you'll be able to play detective and modify your program yourself, but don't be scared or worried if you run into some of these. There's help out there to get you back on track physically and mentally with your exercise goals!

Returning to Sex

Sex will probably feel different. And at first, depending on hormones and healing, there may be some slight discomfort that requires generous lubrication and easing into intercourse with strategy, but sex should not hurt. Painful sex is never normal at any point in life. Don't settle for the advice that you should drink some wine, take a bath, and try to relax a little. Don't settle for the advice that you should just push through and it will get better with time. There may be multiple physical and emotional components at play here.

- Physical elements: scar tissue, healing of muscles/tissue, hormones, tight muscles

- Nervous system and emotional components: guarding of the body from trauma experienced during labor and birth, guarding against the previous time you've tried sex that became painful, and getting comfortable with your new body

If your body perceives that something will be painful, regardless of whether there is actual tissue damage, it will most likely be painful. This chapter will cover advice on how you can get comfortable with your vulva and vagina yourself and with your partner. Just like with return to exercise, the progression you move through will be based on listening to your own body and what it's ready for. Consider seeking out help with a pelvic floor PT, postnatal specialists, and mental health/sex therapists to deal with the various components of your recovery. Also, consider lube!

Here are some examples of how you can ease back into intimacy with your partner. Choose ways that feel comfortable and appropriate for your goals. Often, our lack of awareness, comfort, and confidence in knowing this part of our body may contribute to fear, pain, and tension we feel.

Feeling yourself

Next time you're in the shower or have some time to lie down in a relaxed position, start by feeling your abdominal and pelvic region. Simply begin with the goal of feeling the tissues and muscles on the outside. If you had a cesarean birth, start to feel your lower abdomen and work on making peace with touching this area. For some this may be easy. For others, it's extremely triggering. The next chapter will cover scar tissue in more detail. If you're not ready to touch your scars yet, skip this part. Feel around the rest of your belly. Feel the skin, the muscles, the stretch marks. Get comfortable with your own hands touching your body. Move on to your pelvic area. Touch your vulva. Feel the labia majora and the labia minora and the clitoris. Feel your way around externally and see if there are any painful areas. If so, work on gentle touching that area in a way that does not cause pain. Use gentle touch in a slow, intentional way to increase your positive experience in self-exploration rather than pushing through pain.

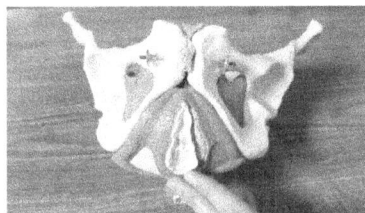

Progress by starting to feel internally. Do so gently. Pretend your vaginal opening is a clock with 12:00 being up towards the urethra/clitoris and 6:00 being towards the anus. Begin by slowly inserting one finger into your vagina towards the 6:00 position. Hold there for a bit and simply sense how it feels. Slowly move your finger towards the 3:00 position, then back to the 6:00, and then toward the 9:00 position. Take your time and try to make this a positive or at least neutral experience. Do not push into pain. Take full breaths as you're doing this and think positive thoughts.

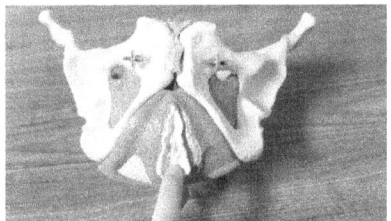

Advance to feel deeper and/or with more speed. Continue to feel in different directions and depths of your vagina. Use different pressures. Feel your pelvic floor muscles internally: contract, relax, and lengthen. Feel your breath gently expand and contract these muscles at a low level naturally. Notice if there are any areas that feel tight or painful and slowly work to bring gentle touch and release to those areas.

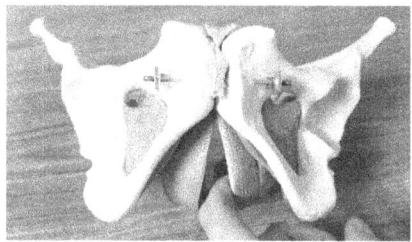

Continue to touch and feel internally and externally in any ways that you may encounter during sexual intercourse. Use this time to make peace with your body and experience physically and mentally. Note if there are certain areas that you will want to be careful and mindful of while returning to intercourse with your partner. Only pursue this exercise as a positive, pain-free experience. Other ways some women find helpful to advance at this point is using a dilator, wand, or sex toys at this point as progression to partner intimacy. Vibration has been shown to help with healing tissue and scars.

Sex and other forms of intimacy

When you feel ready and want to begin being intimate with your partner, have an open conversation about going slowly and speaking up if something doesn't feel right. You may not jump right back into positions or speeds you were used to previously. There may be different positions that are less painful and allow for you to feel more in control of the depth of penetration. There are lots of options as you heal physically and emotionally. As hormones settle back down and you work through the above steps, you should be able to return to sex pain free.

The same way you've worked through touching yourself slowly and intentionally may be something you want to work through with your partner. You may choose to start with external stimulation rather than any forms of penetration if that feels right for you. The more open and honest you can be, your partner can help you into making this a positive, pain-free activity you'll continue to enjoy in the long run. Don't put pressure on yourself to orgasm right away. Find ways to reach the orgasm externally with the clitoris rather than pushing through anything (friction, speed, positions, length of time) you're not ready for it internally.

Again, you should not push through pain. There are specific ways a pelvic floor PT can help you postpartum to work through the physical things at play. A PT can help you better understand how the nervous system and brain is responding in a protective way and how to work through that. Considering talking with a medical provider about hormone contribution if these methods are not helping dryness.

Every woman will get back to sex at different rates based on healing, hormones, and sex drive. Give yourself time and grace to connect with your pelvic floor muscles, breath, vulva, vagina, clitoris, and abdomen. You are beautiful and resilient. You've got this!

Remember What Worked Before

Along with returning to normalcy, you should remind yourself of the things you did to get a slim figure before your pregnancy. As with food, we need to remember what we did activity-wise pre-pregnancy. If that body is the body we are striving for, then we obviously were doing something right before.

With exercise, you don't need to start some totally new and outrageous workout regimen. Using our five-mile run example, the person obviously liked to jog before they got pregnant. So why stop that now? If running was the cardiovascular exercise of choice before the pregnancy, it should also be the exercise of choice after the pregnancy. To beat a dead horse, you don't need to completely start from the beginning. There was a pre-pregnancy process that worked. So, what else did you do? Perhaps you did a lot of bike riding or yoga. Returning to not only what worked in the past but also what you enjoyed in the past will be an easier transition than starting an entirely new and foreign exercise plan.

To be clear, this does not mean that it will be very easy to transition back into the exercises you did in the past. After going through a nine-month pregnancy where your body goes through some major alterations, it may be hard to get back in the groove. So, while some of the details of your activity may need to change, the basics of your approach shouldn't change. For instance, you used to ride your bicycle to work. Your work is about five miles away. Shortly after the pregnancy, you may want to get back to riding your bicycle to work. But this is a big task to undertake immediately following childbirth. So, while bike riding is the right general exercise for you, the distance will not immediately match your expectations. And that's okay. As with short-term goal setting, you need to know your limitations. Begin riding your bicycle again and slowly you will return to cardiovascular shape. It is ultimately a smoother move from no exercise to some exercise if you have accomplished and enjoyed that activity in the past.

Body and Fitness

Hormones

Hormones can cause havoc on losing the baby weight, and demolish our willingness to get motivated. Even though we may not feel great all the time, doesn't mean we cannot use the hormonal shift to our advantage. Some people call it, "Running off the crazy," or "Ridding the rage." Whatever you do, you cannot keep all of those raw emotions locked inside of your psyche and body. Keep telling yourself that working out is the only way to keep yourself and your family safe from the hormones.

Hormones will go up and down, but there is a sudden shift right after the baby is born, and also when you wean from breastfeeding. Try not to panic, but take precautions and talk to a healthcare professional if you need to. Yoga, deep breathing meditation, stretching, and working out will help. Make sure to have a loved one available to watch the baby if post-partum depression happens. The body needs time to adjust and recover from those hormonal shifts. You're not alone in these issues, so don't be afraid to talk to family or reach out to your doctor for help.

Realizing what is happening to our bodies, will only empower you. Embrace the changes with hormones. Take it as a challenge to overcome. Giving birth to your baby was no easy feat, so losing the baby weight will not be easy either. The only kind of work that is worth doing is hard-work. It is described as "hard" for a reason, and every step of this process will be a reason to celebrate your awesomeness.

Importance of Sleep

Welcome to motherhood; let the lack of sleep begin. It is truly amazing how mothers can feed a baby every 2-3 hours, and survive on minimal sleep. Sleep really is important in many ways, but especially when losing the baby weight. In the first year, give yourself time to adapt to the new sleep routine required for your individual baby's needs. However, the more sleep you give yourself, the better you will be able to operate.

There are many ways to get your allotted eight hours of sleep, so don't try to do this all on your own. If you are a single mom, reach out to your friends and family or someone you trust to help you get caught up on sleep. It will get easier once the baby is not feeding so often, but throughout the process sleep is very important and is imperative to weight loss.

Anytime you feel overwhelmed or behind on chores, do not beat yourself up about it. Stop what you're doing, take a deep breath or stretch, and write down 3-5 chores that need to be done that day. Most mothers know that everything changes when having a baby, but don't fret -YOU CAN AND WILL GET IT ALL DONE! Worrying about the number of errands and chores that need to be done can cause insomnia; therefore, worrying about it does nothing but hurt you.

Each day, write down those 3-5 errands or chores that need to be done (priorities first,) and cross them off as you complete them. Please try to not lose sleep over not getting everything done. Your baby is the priority now, so strategize to get chores done, and not lose sleep about it. Writing things down when you remember is helpful; and also hanging lists up where you can see them is a must- such as the refrigerator.

The topic of Caffeine is a sensitive subject for most people, but you will sleep much more restful when eliminating it from your diet. Most people think they need their caffeine boost to function; but health care studies show that it is a very bad choice on your body. Not to mention, it will negatively affect your body's natural sleeping routine.

If you are consuming Caffeine while pregnant or while breastfeeding, the baby is affected in more severe ways; because the baby's organs are not fully developed yet. Caffeine can cause the baby to develop heart troubles and/or other traumatic health issues. It is serious and should not be in your diet, much less your tiny baby's diet.

Do your own research, and don't rely on a chemical to boost your energy. Rely on natural energy boosting foods, and your body's renewable energy cycle. Doing so will help your body to regulate healthy sleep patterns; thus, providing the best sleep possible to recover and renew for top performance.

Takes Time to Recover

Whether the birth was natural, VBAC (vaginal birth after C-section), or C-section every mother needs time to recover. Therefore, there's no need to rush the process of getting back into a skimpy bikini overnight. The body is an amazing creation, and there is a reason for every step towards recovery.

Mothers gain weight during pregnancy because after delivery the body needs extra fuel to produce milk, supply energy for sleep deprivation, rearrange the body's organs back in normal position, and for many other recovery reasons. It can take about a year to drop the baby weight, naturally, and totally recover from the trauma of giving birth.

My advice is to enjoy the process of recovery, and being a new mommy! Try to be present and in the moment every day. Your baby needs you to be happy, loving, and calm. Every day is a blessing and a joy;

therefore, be grateful, and don't worry the weight will come off in due time! All you have to do is stick to the plan, and enjoy your life in the meantime.

C-section Recovery Techniques

**If you're already passed this stage of recovery, feel free to skip ahead.

Keeping your stress level down is key with any serious surgery recovery, and a cesarean section (C-Section) is no different. However, dealing with pain can cause unwanted stress. It's normal to have pain up to two weeks after delivery, and your doctor will most likely prescribe anti-inflammatory medication, or even stronger painkillers. Everybody's pain tolerance is different, so you must do what makes you comfortable. Also, take probiotics to build back up the healthy bacteria in your gut. Antibiotics given during surgery will likely get your body's natural flora off track; which can cause diarrhea and hamper immunity.

Eating right is also key to healing. Focus on eating anti-inflammatory foods that are high in vitamin C; such as, berries, broccoli, and kale. Vitamin C repairs tissues by supporting the production of collagen. Also, eat foods rich in omega-3 fatty acids like nuts and seeds are also inflammatory. Limit red meat- which is inflammatory. Chicken and Salmon are better choices, because they have amino acids which form proteins to repair tissues in the body.

To prevent constipation after surgery: eat fiber-rich foods, drink 100+ ounces of water, prune juice (or prunes), and ask your doctor about a stool softener. Pregnancy hormones, combined with pain killers will most likely lead to constipation. Straining can put pressure on the incision, and healing abdominal muscles- causing pain and discomfort. Also, try a toilet stool (Squatty Putty) or prop your feet on yoga blocks which will straighten the colorectal angle

Breastfeed with support by sitting up straight, and bring your baby close to you. Leaning forward will limit the amount of oxygen the body consumes (also bad for the neck as it strains it,) which will lead to fatigue and will prevent you from retaining the transverse abdominis muscles and fascia (the muscles responsible for holding your abs together.) By the way, whatever position you hold yourself (posture) is the way the body learns and adapts to. Good posture leads to a stronger body- especially when healing.

Things to avoid for the first 8 weeks of recovery: the abdominal binder is usually given to mothers to help with pain, but the binder will take over for the abdominal muscles- preventing the muscles from recovering. A binder will also put added pressure on pelvic organs, causing urinary incontinence. Try a graduated compression undergarment instead that will ease the pain and swelling without the other problems.

Avoid lifting anything heavy, and allow your spouse or family to help with cleaning your home. Each doctor may give a specific weight limitation on lifting, but it is usually no more than the weight of your baby. Ask for help, especially if you're in pain. Ease back into sex, and your doctor may tell you to wait for up to 8 weeks. Intercourse is more likely to be painful after a C-section delivery.

Lastly, avoid crunches because any abdominal muscle workout before the tissues are fully repaired can lead to hernia. There are 7 layers of tissue cut or disturbed during the C-section surgery, and the body needs to repair and recover fully prior to crunches. Consult your doctor about when he advises to begin an abdominal workout. Sometimes doctors will allow plank or bridge core strength training sooner than crunches, but it is always wise to ask first. Better to be safe than in pain.

Vaginal Birth and VBAC Recovery

There are some similarities in recovering from a natural birth compared to a C-section. Some swelling will likely occur, so use the ice-packs the nurse provides to soothe. Do not place directly onto the sensitive skin without protective fabric, and only leave on for up to 15 minutes.

Unfortunately, hemorrhoids usually happen so gently wipe with a Witch Hazel Astringent pad (Tucks) to soothe and relieve. They are also approved for use on vaginal tissue. Similar to the C-section recovery about constipation: try not to strain, and keep drinking water and/or stool softeners until it passes.

If you experienced tearing or an episiotomy, keep the wound clean and allow your body to recover before high impact exercise or movement. Even sitting on the toilet can be tortuous, so finding the most comfortable position while sitting is important. If possible, do not allow yourself to be in pain, and be sure to ask for help when you need it.

Lastly, be sure to do Kegel exercises: which is the tightening of the pelvic muscles. As long as you're not in pain, work on these exercises every day. Just tighten your pelvic muscles, hold for 3 seconds, and then relax for 3 seconds. Start with 3 seconds and then add 1 second each week until you can squeeze and hold for 10 seconds.

Home Workout versus Gym

Everyone is different when finding what motivates them to workout. Some people have great, challenging routines they execute from their homes; while others enjoy going to the gym. Once everything in your life is organized and beaming with promise: adding a working out routine towards your fitness goals will only enhance the happiness!

We must find our purpose that will keep us motivated to work out. Similar to the motivation of a bride-to-be -working out to fit into her perfect wedding dress; or knowing that everything in our life will function better when we are stronger and fit. Find your purpose to why you're getting fit: your baby, looking good in skinny jeans, to feel alive and happy every day, marathon challenges, charity events, and you may have to reset your purpose frequently. Whatever drives you to work hard, is the goal and purpose for our lives.

If you decide to workout at home, be sure to have some good equipment or quality/effective routines available on DVDs for exercise. There are exercise bands, dumbbells, kettle bells, bosa ball, weight bags, and you can even use chairs for various exercises too. People can get creative at home, but just don't allow yourself to get distracted. It is easy to do when the baby cries, or your spouse asks you a question. Give yourself 30 minutes to an hour, put your music on, and focus on your routine.

Lastly, be sure to keep an eye on your caloric intake while working out and breastfeeding. Take care of yourself by making sure you have adequate fuel for your baby, and to compensate for your workout routine. For example, if you burn 400 calories a day from breastfeeding, and another 400 at the gym- be sure to eat the appropriate caloric intake for your Body Mass Index, plus your baby's needs. Remember, like a car, we have to provide our bodies with healthy/ adequate fuel for optimal performance!

Support

I touched on this subject briefly within other categories, but it is important enough to warrant its own discussion. There is almost no chance for success if you plan to approach this process entirely on your own. If the mental aspect of achieving your goals is the most important element (and I firmly believe that it is), then you need to be sure that you are properly supported as you attempt to get back your pre-pregnancy body.

It is easy to say that you should lean on your husband or partner during this time. And honestly, this is the best scenario. But it's also not feasible for everybody. Not everybody has another parent there going through the same things that they are. Most people, however, do have at least one good friend or a family member on whom they can lean. Having the proper support is crucial for so many reasons. Firstly, you will face challenges throughout this process. That is inevitable. Nobody undertakes a weight loss journey and faces no adversity whatsoever. But what you do when you face adversity is the important thing. If you are alone, you are far more likely to give up when met with challenges. There are two reasons for this. Firstly, as we briefly discussed earlier, human beings are far less likely to want to let somebody else down than to let themselves down. In other words, if somebody else knows what you're going through and what your ultimate goals are, they will, simply by having that knowledge, hold you accountable. They may not even need to say anything the least bit motivational. Simply by them knowing what you're attempting to do with help keep you on track. We don't like letting other people down, even if it pertains only to our own goals. If we tell somebody that we are going to accomplish something, we are more likely to do it than if we keep it to ourselves. That is just social science. Secondly, and maybe more importantly, you simply have somebody to talk to. Internalizing your problems is almost never beneficial. It is too easy to stew on mistakes and hiccups when you sit and think about things on your own. When you talk them out, however, especially with somebody who cares about you, you realize that the problems are not as big of a deal as you originally thought, or maybe that the other person has even faced similar challenges and has some thoughtful advice on the topic. Either way, letting out your emotions, goals, fears, failures, and successes is very healthy in the process toward weight loss.

Plus-Sized Moms: Lose Baby Weight Fast

Some supermodels famously fail to gain weight during pregnancy. Former Spice Girl and soccer superstar David Beckham's wife Victoria Beckham told the press that her weight gain while she was pregnant with their fourth child, Harper, was less than a beer belly. Entrepreneur and reality TV star Ivanka Trump posed for Playboy during her pregnancy. In 2010, television personality Bethany Frankel reported she had lost 31 pounds (13.5 kilograms) in less than month after giving birth.

Most mothers, however, definitely show weight gain during pregnancy and take a lot longer than a month to get back to normal — and probably have healthier children. New mothers who don't have housekeepers, trainers, drivers, and chefs have a lot more to do than just to lose weight, but even ordinary moms usually can get their figures back, eventually.

Here are 10 tips for losing weight after baby is born:

1.   Forget about dieting until your baby is six weeks old.

The first step in weight loss for most new mothers is to be absolutely sure you aren't still eating for two. It is more important not to gain weight, at least for the first few weeks, than it is to lose it.

2.   Breastfeed your baby as often as possible.

Breastfeeding confers babies with distinct advantages. Breast milk is almost the perfect food for a growing child. (It may be deficient in vitamin D, but getting sun, without sunburn, takes care of that deficiency.) Breastfed babies are less likely to develop allergies and eczema, and they gain their mothers' immune resistance to many diseases. Babies who are fed mother's milk are less likely to be obese as adults and score higher on IQ tests, Moreover, mothers who breastfeed their babies lose pregnancy weight faster.

The effects of breastfeeding on weight loss can be dramatic. In one study, mothers who breastfed, on average, weighed 2 pounds (1 kilo) less three months after giving birth than they did before they got pregnant. Even when mothers have trouble adjusting their eating habits after giving birth, breastfeeding helps prevent continuing weight gain.

3.   Get more exercise than just carrying baby around.

Taking care of a baby can be a real workout in itself, but it doesn't exercise all the muscle groups. To prevent injuries and to encourage all your muscles to burn calories, get at least a little baby-free exercise time. A baby-friendly gym can be a place to reconnect with adult friends, especially at "mommy and me" classes offered at many gyms. As your child gets older, a little time with babysitters at the gym will help with the development of social skills.

How much exercise is enough? Most experts recommend 150 minutes (two and one-half hours) a week, ideally about half an hour at a time, five times a week. If it is simply impossible to find an uninterrupted half hour, exercise 10 minutes at a time 15 times a week, any time exercise is possible. If you have had few opportunities to do any kind of exercise during pregnancy, start out with very easy resistance exercise. Even lifting a couple of soup cans can rebuild muscles, and muscles burn fat and store sugars to improve not just weight but also general health. Looking for ways to get a few minutes of exercise? Ease back into exercise with simple moves that include your baby in your routine:

Dance! Put on your favorite dance music and do a little dance for your baby. One mother report that she puts on cheesy 80's disco music and does disco dancing while baby watches.

Try baby-cise. Carefully balance your baby as you do sit-ups, squats, and arm lifts.

Move the diaper changing station upstairs, downstairs, or any place you have to take a few extra steps to take care of your baby.

4. Eat fish, or take fish oil or microalgae oil.

Fish is a superfood for new moms. Cold-water fish is a great source of the essential fatty acids eicosatetraenoic acid (EPA), which minimizes inflammation, and docosahexaenoic acid (DHA), which builds healthy nerves. Part of mother's DHA and EPA finds its way to breast milk, and helps the baby develop faster and smarter; results continuing even years after breastfeeding have been discontinued. EPA also reduces inflammation in fat tissues and allows greater circulation of fluids that would otherwise be trapped inside. Getting rid of these fluids takes off weight without exercise or calorie restriction.

Three 3-1/2 oz (100 gram) servings of fish every week is enough. If you don't care for fish, take fish oil or microalgae oil--but avoid alcohol. Alcohol damages EPA and DHA so that they cannot exert their beneficial health effects, and can even cause atherosclerosis.

5. Avoid (or, even better, eliminate) sugary foods.

Sugar-sweetened soft drinks, sweet tea, sugar-sweetened fruit juice, snack cakes, cookies, ice cream, and candy do not add calories that can be turned into fat. They also increase inflammation that can add water weight. Especially if you notice achy joints after eating sugar, you need to avoid sugar in all its forms.

6. Hide problem foods.

If you let yourself eat whole bags of chips or packages of cookies while you were pregnant, put your most tempting goodies out of sight to keep them out of mind. Many mothers keep snacks in the freezer, preferably a freezer in a garage or a basement, requiring additional effort to eat them. Save the foods you know you shouldn't eat but you really want to eat for those times when the urge is overwhelming. Then eat slowly, and less than you really want. Snack foods and desserts usually keep for later.

7. If you can't cut back a lot, cut back a little.

If you usually eat cheese on meat in your sandwich, skip the cheese and just eat the meat. If you usually eat two sandwiches at a meal, eat one. Avoid the chips and candy aisles when you go grocery shopping. If you just have to have a dessert, try a pudding cup or a 100-calorie package of cookies or nuts.

8. Use a stroller.

Take your baby outside in a stroller every day the weather permits. You get exercise, and your baby gets fresh air and vitamin D. Taking a different route every day, as long as the neighborhood is safe, helps you burn more calories. It takes more energy to walk along a new route than along an old one.

9.   Play with the pooch.

Walking the family dog, and exercising with the dog, burns calories — and is great for the dog.

10. Toss the take-out menus.

Take-out meals come in larger portions than you would probably cook for yourself. To keep customers happy, restaurants make sure to include fat, salt, and flavorings that encourage you to eat more, more, more. Cook low-fat, easy meals for yourself, and limit take-out and sit-down restaurant meals to just once or twice a month, and avoid fast food and Starbucks, too.

The first year of your baby's life is likely to be a very busy time. It can be almost impossible to juggle the demands of taking care of your child with the demands of dieting. These ten tips can help you take off extra weight without the stress of dieting.

HEALING YOUR VAGINA NATURALLY

During pregnancy many women experience swelling, discharge, varicosities (veins popping out), and other symptoms that affect the vagina. Your vagina is sore, swollen, and in serious need of some TLC. Following vaginal birth, pain, swelling, bleeding, and overall discomfort is par for the course.

The time it will take for your vaginal tissue to heal and recover is variable depending on the extent of the trauma—including if you had a tear or episiotomy. Caring for your body using natural remedies will not only help you recover more quickly, but will also decrease the amount of discomfort you are experiencing.

Early Vaginal Bleeding

Lochia is the medical term for the vaginal bleeding that occurs postpartum. It is normal and you will often see many clots, which can vary in size.

The bleeding generally transitions from red to brown and eventually becomes a yellow or clear discharge. For many women, the discharge will be gone by 4 weeks postpartum, but some may have discharge up to 8 weeks.

If you experience new onset of heavy bleeding or large clots after the discharge has stopped or feel concerned about the discharge, be sure to speak with your healthcare provider.

Do not use a tampon, menstrual cup or insert anything into the vagina during your first 6 weeks postpartum. Instead, opt for organic pads and change often to avoid vaginal irritation.

Natural Remedies to Heal and Soothe Sore Tissue

Sitz Baths. Traditional sitz baths, which consist of having one tub with cold water and another with warm that you alternate between, are the most ideal, but you may not have easy access to a bathtub or even have the energy to set up a sitz bath. Because of this, I recommend a modified postpartum sitz bath utilizing herbs to encourage tissue healing and soothe the area.

Postpartum Sitz Bath. Place the herbs directly into a muslin bag and immerse the bag in the hot water of the bath. To do this, run the bath water with only hot water, place the muslin bag and one cup of Epsom salt into the bath water and allow to steep. Once the water has reached a comfortable temperature you can get into the bathtub. Remember, you only need enough to cover the genital area, so if you're not up for a full bath, just place a small amount of water in the bathtub.

Herbs for Sitz Baths

- Calendula flower: antimicrobial, soothing, anti-inflammatory

- Rosemary leaves: antimicrobial

- Comfrey leaves: promotes tissue healing

- Lavender flower: antimicrobial, relaxing

- Thyme leaves: antimicrobial

- Uva ursi berry: antimicrobial

- Shepherd's purse leaf: hemostatic (stops blood flow)

- Yarrow: antibacterial, antifungal, hemostatic

Choose ½ cup each of four to six of these herbs and place in a large bowl to mix well. Place the herbs in a large Mason jar and store in a cool dry place. When ready to use, take ¼ cup of the mixture and place in a muslin bag for your bath or use any of the following methods.

It's important that you do not apply too much heat or stay immersed in hot water for too long as it can create pelvic stagnation. Consider ending the bath after 20 minutes of heat or when the water cools.

To increase circulation and promote healing, end the bath with a cold compress placed directly on the genital area for 10 minutes or run cool water over the vaginal tissue for 30 seconds.

Making a Topical Tea. Bring two quarts of water to a boil. Add one cup of herbs and remove from the heat. Cover and allow to sit for 20 minutes. Strain and allow to cool. Use as a rinse at the end of your shower.

Note: The herbal mixture will keep at room temperature for about 6-8 hours, in the fridge for three days. Do not take internally.

Herbal Peri Bottle Rinse. Place cooled Topical Tea (see above) in a peri bottle. To use, apply a stream of fluid from the peri bottle to the vaginal tissue during urination and following using the restroom.

Herbal Cold Compresses. Apply the Topical Tea to organic pads or reusable organic cloth and place in the freezer. Apply these cold packs to the vaginal tissue, either allowing them to warm or removing after 10-15 minutes. Take care not to over-apply cold compresses.

Apply as often as you find necessary for the first three to seven days.

What if I'm birthing in a hospital?

You can make individual muslin herb bags prior to delivery and store them in plastic bags or storage containers to keep in your hospital bag. In a pinch, you can place them in a basin of very hot water and use both the water and muslin herb bag to cleanse the area once the water has reached a comfortable temperature.

When to talk to your healthcare provider:

If you've had a major tear, trauma, or an infection, please discuss these therapies with your doctor. They may be contraindicated in early postpartum. Signs of infection include fever, chills, nausea, vomiting, extreme redness, tenderness, foul odor, or pus.

Healing Vaginal Tears & Episiotomy

If you've experienced severe tearing, ask your doctor about using a topical antimicrobial following bowel movements and urination. Sometimes, a simple water and iodine solution will be recommended if you don't have an iodine allergy

Keeping a clean peri bottle next to the sink to be used when you void will help decrease discomfort. Fill the peri bottle with warm water and express the water onto the urethra during urination to help dilute the urine to make the sensitive tissue more comfortable.

You can also use the herbal sitz baths wash solution in the peri bottle.

Using the same principles and techniques to heal the vaginal tissue as previously discussed will also improve the healing of tears. Some women have residual pain and discomfort even after the tissue has healed. If this is the case for you, you should consider speaking with your doctor and a pelvic floor physical therapist.

Healing Vulvovaginal Varicosities (Dilated Veins)

During pregnancy there is a great deal of pressure on the pelvis and, as a result, circulation isn't at its best. Many women experience mild dilations of the veins in the vulvar area. It is not uncommon for these to resolve after pregnancy; however, if they become enlarged, hot, or painful after birth please speak with your doctor.

Sitz Baths. Sitz baths using comfrey, yellow dock, plantain and yarrow reduce swelling and relieve discomfort.

Hydrotherapy. Alternating hot and cold hydrotherapy heals the tissue and increases circulation. For new moms, I recommend performing hydrotherapy in the shower. At the end of your shower, turn the water to cool-cold and apply directly to your pelvis and the affected area. If you have a removable shower head, apply the cold water directly to the veins.

Apply warm water for 1 minute followed by cold water for 30 seconds. Repeat for a total of 3 rounds, always ending with cold.

Vitamin E. 400 IU daily, taken internally to promote antioxidant activity and healing of the blood vessels may be used. You may also apply the oil topically to the affected tissue to soothe and aid in healing.

Bioflavonoids. 1,000 mg. daily supports blood vessel integrity to prevent the vein from enlarging further.

Homeopathic Calc Fluor cell salt 6x. 3-5 tabs 3 times daily to stabilize connective tissue.

Preventing Pelvic Organ Prolapse

I recommend that women rest in bed and lay down as often as possible for at least 2 weeks following childbirth. Relaxin, the hormone that allowed your cervix to soften and your hips to widen, can remain in your system up to 6 months after delivery. This is why some women experience joint instability and can be injured with early intense exercise.

Why is it important to minimize time on your feet?

In the beginning, when relaxin is still high, the uterus is heavy, and the pelvic floor muscles are in need of recovery, you are at risk for developing a vaginal and uterine prolapse. The combination of all these factors, plus gravity and the potential overextending yourself can put you at even greater risk.

Refrain from being overly active is the main message I want you to walk away with. Yes, you can grab a snack, use the restroom and engage in very light activity, but in those early weeks really focus on resting as often as possible.

In Chinese medicine they recommend that the feet don't touch the floor for the first 40 days following childbirth. This is a beautiful illustration of the kind of support you'll need in those first weeks after childbirth. Obviously, this is ideal but not always possible.

If you feel heaviness begin to develop in your pelvis, take this as a sign that it is time to rest. Sensations of pressure and bulging are common with pelvic prolapse.

Types of Prolapse:

Cystocele (Anterior Vaginal Wall Prolapse): Herniation of the anterior wall (bellybutton side) of the vagina, with or without dropping of bladder.

Common Symptoms: Urinary incontinence or difficulty with urination.

Rectocele (Posterior Vaginal Wall Prolapse): Herniation of the posterior wall (back side) of the vagina, with or without dropping of rectum.

Common Symptoms: Constipation, fecal incontinence, urgency.

Enterocele: Intestines protrude through or to the vaginal wall.

Common Symptoms: Pelvic fullness, pelvic pain, bulge sensation in the vagina, pain with intercourse, pulling sensation in pelvis that is better with lying down.

Apical Compartment Prolapse: Descent of the uterus or upper portion of the vagina to the opening of the vagina.

Common Symptoms: Urinary incontinence or difficulty with urination, bulge sensation in vagina.

Because the vagina is a continuous organ, it can be difficult to differentiate a prolapse and often there can be an issue with several aspects of the vagina.

Working with a skilled pelvic floor provider to rehabilitate stretched muscles and support the organs of the pelvis will enable your body to heal. Further medical intervention may be necessary and your health care provider can assist you in ensuring you are having the necessary care to heal your body.

Holistic Pelvic Care™ is an internal vaginal massage technique combined with mind-body breath work to heal the pelvic floor physically and energetically. This powerful therapy was developed by Tami Lynn Kent, a women's health physical therapist and author of Wild Feminine.

Vaginal Wind

Vaginal wind or the release of air from the vagina is very common in the early postpartum healing. There's a lot of laxity in the tissue. You passed a human through a very small space—which has weakened your vaginal tone. While it can feel embarrassing, it's nothing to be ashamed of. It's very common. Most women experience it.

Performing Kegels can help you regain tone. You may also consider working with a trained pelvic floor professional to increase your vaginal tone.

Because many women feel embarrassed when there is a release of air from the vagina, you may want to practice exercises or yoga moves at home before you go to a class. For example, audible vaginal gas can be passed when moving from down dog (a yoga pose) into another position, and although completely normal it is far from ideal.

Exercise for the Pelvic Floor (aka vagina rehab)

Traditionally prescribed for urinary incontinence, Kegel exercises are only part of the equation when it comes to rehabbing the vagina. Now, I don't think Kegels are bad, in fact I think working these muscles increases circulation to the pelvis. Increased blood flow and lymphatic (immune system) flow promotes healing while helping your body fight microbes that could cause infection. Performing Kegels early in postpartum can also help you maintain muscle tone and reduce the risk of other complications, such as incontinence or organ prolapse.

But there are a lot of complications that can arise after a small human pass through the vaginal canal—pelvic pain, scar tissue, pain with intercourse, incontinence, vaginal prolapse. I think you get the picture. And many of these symptoms can interfere with day-to-day life and subsequent pregnancies.

How to Perform a Kegel?

The first step in performing a Kegel exercise is to identify the target muscles. There are couple approaches to helping you to identify these muscles. I recommend using the one that makes the most sense to you, but you can certainly try both.

Stopping the Flow of Urine. While urinating, stop the flow midstream by engaging your pelvic floor muscles. This is not the actual exercise, but will help you identify the muscles you want to engage. I recommend only trying this once, maybe twice to avoid increasing the risk of a bladder infection.

Examine Your Vaginal Floor. Insert one lubricated finger into the vagina. Contract the pelvic floor so that you feel the walls of your vagina squeezing inward and upward around your finger.

When you're ready, contract the pelvic floor and imagine you are lifting the vagina towards the crown on the head and hold for at least 2 seconds. Relax the pelvic floor completely and then repeat.

Four Common Kegel Mistakes:

Contracting the Wrong Muscles. When performing a Kegel, the glutes, thighs and abdominal muscles should be relaxed. The focus should be on the pelvic floor.

Pushing Down Instead of Pulling Up. Bearing down, similar to when having a bowel movement, is a common mistake when performing a Kegel. It may be helpful to insert one finger vaginally so you can feel the direction of the contraction.

Forgetting to Release the Contraction. Relaxing completely is as important as the exercise itself. Maintaining the contraction without relaxing can cause the muscles to become over worked and creates too much tension in the muscles, which may lead to pelvic floor dysfunction.

Lack of Consistency. Like all muscles in the body, consistency is necessary for building strength. Don't give up too early!

Sample Exercise for Pelvic Floor:

1. Contract the pelvic floor, lifting the muscles up.

2. Hold for 2-3 seconds.

3. Relax for 2-3 seconds.

4. Repeat for a set of 5-10.

Start slow and take care not to fatigue the muscles. If you are experiencing urinary incontinence, overworking the muscles can make symptoms worse. It is better to start with a few repetitions and build up to more over time. Listen to what your body needs and be gentle in not overdoing the exercise.

Having an experienced practitioner perform myofascial work (soft tissue therapy) with you as an active participant can help alleviate trigger points and allow you to have a more uniform contraction of the muscles. They can also assist you in learning how to properly engage the pelvic floor in day-to-day life.

Not all pelvic floor issues can be solved with Kegels alone. I recommend working with a qualified practitioner to fine tune muscle imbalances and ensure you do not over strengthen the pelvic floor (yes, that happens) in relation to other muscle groups.

I generally recommend women begin pelvic floor therapy after they've been cleared at their 6-week postpartum check-up. Working with an experienced physical therapist or Holistic Pelvic Care™ provider can ensure your pelvic floor gets the attention it needs and long-term complications, such as pelvic pain, can be prevented.

Is a 6-week Check-up Necessary?

You should absolutely have your 6-week checkup with your doctor or midwife following delivery. This is where they check how the tissue is repairing and healing, making sure that there are no signs of infection and that your uterus is healing properly. It's more than just getting a clearance for sex and exercise. While it's important to know whether your body is ready for these activities, it's also important to have other symptoms evaluated at that time.

Labs to Consider Testing Postpartum

Depending on what your birth was like, your current symptoms, healthy history and family history your doctor may want to order labs anywhere from 6 weeks to 3 months postpartum.

Lab	Evaluation
Complete Blood Count (CBC)	Evaluates white blood cells, red blood cells, and screen for anemia.
Ferritin	Evaluates iron stores.
Comprehensive Metabolic Panel (CMP)	Evaluates liver, kidney, and gallbladder function.
Thyroid Panel (TSH, Total T3, Total T4, Free T3, Free T4, Reverse T3)	Evaluates thyroid function and health.
Thyroid Antibodies (Anti-TPO, Anti-Thyroglobulin)	Screens for autoimmune postpartum thyroiditis.

Vitamin D	Determine vitamin D status and evaluate if supplementation is warranted.
B12 and Methylmalonic Acid	Evaluates vitamin B12 status.
Folate	Evaluates folate status.
Homocysteine	Indirect marker of inflammation that also gives insight into B vitamin utilization.
MTHFR Gene	Evaluate if there are underlying genetic issues that may affect mental health, energy utilization and detox pathways.
HgA1C	Marker of blood sugar over a 3-month period. Important if you had gestational diabetes.
CRP and/or ESR	Measurement of inflammation
Salivary Cortisol	Determines function and health of adrenal glands.

Natural Relief for After Birth Pains

After birth pains are normal and they can be pretty extreme for some women. They are the result of your uterus contracting back to its original size, a process known as involution.

These contractions generally begin about 12 hours following delivery and may be as mild as your menstrual cramps or as intense as labor contractions. Each time you nurse in the early days following birth you will also feel these contractions. That is because baby's nursing stimulates the release of oxytocin, often called the "cuddle hormone," which causes contractions and helps return your uterus to its original size, among other things. Another benefit to breastfeeding!

In addition to returning your uterus to its original size, these contractions also prevent excess bleeding, which is why it is important to avoid aspirin. Aspirin thins the blood and can lead to increased bleeding.

If you feel like you need to take something for these contractions, try to avoid acetaminophen or ibuprofen as these have side effects that can impact your health, such as leading to intestinal irritation. Instead keep the following remedies near you when you breastfeed to alleviate pain:

Homeopathic Mag Phos 6C. Take 3-5 pellets every 15 minutes for pain. You may find it helpful to take a dose just before you begin nursing.

Hot Water Bottle. Apply heat up to 20 minutes to the low abdomen. Wrap the outside of the hot water bottle with a towel and avoid making contact with baby.

Cramp Bark (Viburnum opulus) Tincture. Take 2 droppers full just before you nurse. It reduces pain without inhibiting the uterus from shrinking.

Motherwort (Leonurus cardiac) Tincture. Take 2 droppers full up to 4 times daily. Motherwort is a uterine tonic and also eases anxiety, irritability, and supports a healthy heart.

Uterine Massage. Every time before you stand up for the first 3-6 weeks postpartum, massage your uterus. Make your hand into a fist and knead the lower belly. This is a technique that may help decrease the amount of bleeding and help the uterus heal.

Natural Remedies to Heal Urinary Tract Infections

Urgency, frequency, or pain with urination may be a sign of a urinary tract infection (UTI). It is wise to contact your doctor if you experience these symptoms, especially if you have a fever, nausea, back ache, or see blood in your urine. If caught early you may not require an antibiotic. However, if there is any risk of the infection affecting your kidneys you want to act quickly and meet with your doctor, as an antibiotic will be necessary to resolve the infection and protect your kidneys.

Prevention:

- Wear white cotton underwear changed daily

- Use only mild, natural detergents on clothing

- Use non-deodorized, preferably organic, sanitary pads

- Wipe front to back after bowel movement

- Avoid bubble baths

- Shower after swimming

- Avoid tight pants

- Eat lacto-fermented foods 3 times weekly

Natural Treatment of Urinary Tract Infection

Diet: Avoid sugar, alcohol, caffeine, aspartame, and dried fruits until symptoms resolve.

Increase Water Intake: Drink a glass of filtered water every 20 minutes for 2 hours then every hour for 24 hours, except during sleep.

Vitamin C: 1,000 mg 4-5 times daily for two days. Can cause loose stools, so decrease the dose if this occurs. After two days, reduce dose to 500 mg 4-5 times daily for five days.

Cranberry Juice: Drink 4 ounces of unsweetened cranberry juice 4 times daily for 1 week.

Cranberry D-Mannose: 2 capsules twice daily for 1 week.

Homeopathic Remedies:

- Cantharis 30C: Use when there is painful burning with urination.

- Equisetum 30C: Use when there is pain and there's a sensation that the bladder is always full, despite having just urinated.

- Sarsaparilla 30C: Pain at the end of urination, may not be able to void unless done so standing up.

- Berberis 30C: Painful bladder, relieved by urination.

- Staphysagria 30C: UTI comes on after intercourse.

To use Homeopathic remedies: 3-5 pellets 15-minutes away from food every 2-4 hours until symptoms are resolved.

Urinary Incontinence

You sneeze, you pee. You cough, you pee. You pick up your baby … and you pee. It is not only inconvenient, but also embarrassing. And it's also a common symptom following childbirth.

Some women will easily recover and will not experience long-term issues with urinations, while others will go on to experience a daily incontinence or urinary leakage.

Kegels (see How to Perform a Kegel) are one way in which you can strengthen the pelvic floor to reduce or eliminate urinary incontinence. You may also want to consider meeting with a Holistic Pelvic Care™ practitioner or a pelvic floor physical therapist to help you understanding the muscle imbalances that are contributing to your symptoms (Hint: Kegels aren't always enough.)

If you are having trouble with urine leakage, try bending forward at your waist next time you need to cough or sneeze. This will decrease the amount of downward pressure on the pelvic floor.

Natural Healing After a C-Section

I think it is important to acknowledge that there is no shame in having a C-section. Many women, especially those who were planning a natural birth, feel ashamed and sometimes defeated after a C-section, as if they did something wrong because they didn't delivery their baby vaginally. There is no shame in doing whatever it took to bring your baby into this world and to ensure their health and yours, no matter the procedure.

Regardless of the type of delivery, you are a mother and you have a beautiful baby to be grateful for. You're amazing—today and every day.

For most women, a small layer of skin begins to heal over the wound within 48 hours, protecting it from bacterial infections. However, this skin is fragile and easily disrupted. Typically, women are able to shower after the first 48 hours following delivery.

Please contact your health care provider immediately if you experience pain at the site, fever, discharge from the wound, the tissue becomes red or there is an odor present.

Many women find the following tips helpful in healing from a C-Section.

Keep the wound dry and clean. After your showers, gently pat the wound area dry. Avoid clothing, which rubs against the wound site.

Bone Broth. Drink at least one cup daily. Along with being easy to digest, bone broth is rich in minerals and amino acids to aid your body in healing. See recipe.

Grass-fed Gelatin. Consume 2-4 tablespoons daily. Another source of amino acids to support connective tissue healing.

Rest and Sleep. You are recovering from a surgery. Take it slow and allow your body time to heal.

Ask for Help. Get help wherever you can to reduce the need to be up and about.

Anything you can get help with to reduce your need to be up and about will allow your body the much-needed time it needs to rest.

Exercise and Activity

Do NOT skip over this chapter! Don't even think about it. Don't be scared. This is a key chapter to engage with if you want that amazing body! It is not written for the already super fit athletes. It is written for you! You can begin to exercise! You can become fit! You can even be super fit! You can change your body! Everyone has to start somewhere, and here is that place. ...

Let's consider the benefits of exercise

There are many well-documented benefits of exercise. These are worth reviewing in order to remind us that these advantages are broader than simply looking good! Overviewing the benefits of exercise will definitely fuel our level of motivation.

Here are some of the benefits:

Promotes weight loss

Improves your cardiovascular fitness

Improves muscle strength

Reduces risk of heart disease

Reduces risk of diabetes

Increases bone mineral density i.e. stronger bones, and therefore reduces risk of post-menopausal osteoporosis

Increases capacity for daily tasks i.e. increased stamina

Improves body function i.e. coordination and strength, which improve the ability to perform physical tasks (note that the capacity for daily tasks and ability to perform daily tasks are not the same thing).

Lowers health bills

Strengthens immunity (immediately post exercise, your immune system is suppressed, however, in the long term, you will have a much stronger resistance to sickness and diseases).

De-stressing effect

Improves your mood

Helps prevent and promote recovery from postpartum depression

Types of exercise

There are lots of ways to exercise. Most of which are not particularly right or wrong, but some methods are more effective than others. Some people have different preferences too. My general philosophy is to exercise for physical and mental health and longevity, and therefore I chose to do a wide variety of fun activities, alongside a few fundamental aspects that I regard as essential (these can be fun too). It is true that if you are training to run a marathon, you need to run lots. If you are training for a triathlon, you need to include lots of swimming, cycling and running. However, if your focus is to recover from pregnancy and for general fitness, health and happiness, then this chapter is perfect, revealing how best to accomplish this. It will also shortcut your way to having that amazing body you want!

#1 – Include weight training in your program

Incorporating some form of weight training is one of the keys to great health and looking good. An increase in muscle mass will increase your metabolism and thus increase the body's fat burning capabilities. Note that 1lb of muscle in your body burns around 50 calories per day (doing nothing, just living!) In comparison, 1lb of fat burns only about 4 calories per day. Therefore, if you have more muscle you will be burning off significantly more calories throughout each and every day. Eventually this calorie burning process burns off excess fat. Weight training will also give you a better body shape. Contrary to what many believe, you will not look larger or "chunky" by increasing muscle mass. In fact, you will look leaner as your body proportions will be more balanced.

There are many benefits of weight training, some of which are listed above in the benefits of general exercise. I would also like to highlight some specific benefits of weight training which impact how you look and feel:

Stronger body

Increased metabolism (increased fat burning capabilities)

Reduced risk of injury (stronger muscles and joints)

Reduced risk of heart disease and diabetes

Better balance and coordination

Better body shape

It is beneficial to avoid a narrow exercise program where you only include running or another type of cardiovascular exercise. For optimal body composition, this is not ideal due to the catabolic effect of cardiovascular exercise. This simply means doing cardio work alone burns muscle as well as fat, so your overall body composition will be out of balance and you will not gain the tone and shape you desire. Remember, having muscles give a toned look and great shape! The added bonus is that muscle helps burn fat! Furthermore, if you follow a limited exercise program including only cardiovascular exercise, you will suppress the body's production of testosterone, which is needed for everyday function.

During a workout, aerobic exercise may burn more calories than weight training, yet weight training builds more lean muscle mass. These muscles then continue to burn calories even when your body is at rest. Increasing your lean muscle mass therefore increases your body's ability to burn calories both during and after your workout. Clearly, it is best to include both types of exercise in your program. Include exercises that target both your upper and lower body, choosing a weight that allows you to perform one set of 10 to 15 repetitions of each exercise. Aim to do some strength training two or more times per week. It does not necessarily have to be a separate session. I find it works best when I incorporate weight bearing exercise within an aerobic or anaerobic session. Aim to increase the number of sets and the weight you lift as your strength improves.

#2 Include aerobic AND anaerobic exercise in your program

Aerobic exercise is low intensity exercise where you maintain the same pace or intensity for a prolonged period of time. Examples include running, swimming, walking, and cycling, to mention just a few. The benefits of aerobic exercise are numerous, but in particular strengthening your heart and lungs. Anaerobic exercise is where the intensity of the exercise is too high to maintain for a long period of time, thus leading you take moments of rest between work 'intervals. Typically, you would work at a high intensity for 30-60 seconds with a 30-60 second break between these intervals, although these parameters can be varied. High intensity intervals can be performed running, rowing, swimming, cycling, with bodyweight exercises (circuits) or with weights. Like aerobic training, this form of training also works your heart and lungs well too. For example if you do a 10 minute warm-up, 6 sets of 30 seconds of work and 30 seconds of rest, rest for 2 minutes and do 3-4 blocks of this, each with a 2 minute rest period between, followed by a 10 minute cool down, your heart rate has been elevated for 50 minutes and your lungs will have had a great work out! This type of training is best for moms trying to lose baby weight ... the major benefit of anaerobic training being rapid and effective weight loss! Scientific research has revealed this to be the best form of weight loss training. Anaerobic training is even more effective if the interval training involves resistance provided by weights, medicine balls, sand bags or other types of implements, as opposed to performing intervals without resistance, for example running or cycling.

Sports such as soccer, hockey, netball and so on, contain both aerobic and anaerobic elements, and therefore are a great way to exercise and lose weight.

Bodyweight circuits, body pump and other similar exercise classes are good examples of aerobic sessions, which contain elements of anaerobic work interspersed throughout too. However, contrary to the understanding of many, you do not always need a gym or leisure center to provide exercise like this. With a little creativity and imagination, it is possible to set your own sessions up at home or in the garden! Believe me, I meet a friend once week and we enjoy a great work out in the garden together. We get the music on, get some basic pieces of equipment ready, and hope that the sun shines!

Aerobic exercise burns calories, helps you regain some basic muscle strength and builds stamina. Start slowly with low-impact, calorie-burning exercises such as swimming, cycling, walking and the X-trainer. Experts recommend at least 30 minutes of physical activity five or more days a week for everyone. Obviously, as a new mom, you need to work towards this (more on progression later). It is quite easy for new moms to get plenty aerobic exercise. Simply taking your baby out in the pushchair for a daily brisk walk is perfect! Following an aerobics or dance DVD at home or attending a group fitness class for an effective aerobic workout will add variety. Build duration and intensity to your workouts as your strength and stamina improve.

#3 Exercise that improves function / General Conditioning

There are many exercises that can be done which have a positive impact on balance, stability, and body function. These exercises are sometimes done in exercise classes and can also be found on exercise DVD's. They work through fundamental movements that the body should be able to do, challenging balance and coordination. Examples of these types of exercises include lunges, squats, single leg squats, core exercises, overhead squats and arabesques. They give the body a level of robustness that lays a foundation for more rigorous forms of exercise, including weight training and high intensity intervals. These exercises also provide a strong base of conditioning for many popular activities such as sailing, canoeing, skiing, rock climbing and for participating in competitive sports such as netball, hockey, soccer, volleyball or dance. They strengthen the muscles, tendons, ligaments, connective tissue, and stabilize the joints. As a result, risk of injury is reduced.

#4 Exercise that improves Posture & Flexibility

If the types of exercises mentioned above are performed in a technically correct manner, they provide two additional benefits. Firstly, they improve posture, allowing you to stand up straight and be well aligned from the tip of your head to the soles of your feet. This is important for long term health and mobility and can help to eradicate back pain or other forms of chronic pain. Evidently, good posture makes you look better and feel more confident. It even communicates a sense of confidence to others, which can be useful!

Secondly, if these exercises are performed through a full range of motion, as they should be, they will help to improve your joint mobility and flexibility. Joint mobility, along with good posture, unfortunately naturally decline with age, and therefore working on both of these areas becomes even more important. Many breastfeeding moms find they round their shoulders a lot whilst breastfeeding. This can lead to neck and shoulder pain and improper posture. Therefore, try to be aware of your posture during feeding. Find a comfortable and supported position where you do not have to hunch forward!

#5 General activity

Physical activity is important for health and longevity. Consequently, it is important to be involved in a wide range of activities to strengthen different muscle groups and different aspects of fitness. As you include the fundamental principles of exercise explained in this chapter, it doesn't really matter what else you do, as long as you remain active. Being active plays a huge role in overall fitness and calories burned and for that reason it is good to make sure you are active in as many areas of your life as possible. Avoid living a sedentary life surrounding the exceptional moments when you drag yourself out for a jog, or go to your local leisure center to do an aerobics class. You need to be active throughout the day. When possible and realistic try walking rather than taking the car, take the stairs instead of the escalator, sit less and stand more, and play with your children in the park instead of sitting on a bench watching them play.

Principles of exercise

One of the most commonly asked questions is "how soon after the baby is born can I start exercising?" To answer this question, it really depends on how long it takes for you to heal and feel ready to exercise again. Usually, it is 5 to 6 weeks before you feel like doing any intense exercise. And this, ideally, should be only done following a medical check. However, there are gentle exercises you can do from day one! I want to highlight the importance of doing pelvic floor exercises. I know many women skip these, not understanding the importance of them. I guess most people think that these exercises make no difference to their appearance or to the way they feel and therefore lack the motivation to do them. To explain, the pelvic floor muscles get weaker as you get older and especially following pregnancy. Weakened, they can cause problems including urinary incontinence and reduced sensitivity during sex. This is a new chapter of your life, so take this opportunity to start afresh. Be positive, be in control, and value yourself and your future. This is the very beginning of the new you. View these exercises as the first steps of your life journey with exercise being part of your lifestyle. You can't actually do much more on the first few days anyway, so please, just do them. By performing them you begin the reactivation of your core muscles, upon which, you will build. Let's be honest, it may be boring, but surely right now the thrill of having a new baby will get you through these dull moments of the day! You will notice improvement quickly, and believe me, the stronger they are the better for your future involvement in activities that involve any running or dancing or jumping! As a keen netball player (which requires lots of jumping and stretching) I experienced the concern of weakened pelvic floor muscles and so I worked on them!!! As you recover from labor and later down the line, you can do the star jump test to see if you need to continue to work on them!

I would encourage you to start going for short walks as soon as you feel able to do i.e. in the first week after birth. A little bit of fresh air every day is good for you both physically and mentally. A short walk should leave you feeling refreshed and energized, and not exhausted. You can start with just a five-minute walk and build on this over time. Some moms manage to accumulate hours of walking in a day, especially when the baby sleeps well with the motion of the pushchair! Simply walking creates an excellent base level of fitness. As your fitness improves you will be able to extend the amount of time you walk and increase the pace.

In these first few weeks, your focus of exercise should not be weight loss, but merely getting out and about, being mobile, getting fresh air, catching up with friends and for your body to begin to feel normal again. If you are breastfeeding, you will certainly need energy to establish a good milk supply and therefore intense exercise at this point is not advisable. Even in the first few weeks many women notice some early weight loss. Some of this weight loss is due to the body getting rid of extra fluid gained during pregnancy, but some will also be fat loss. Experts suggest that a woman's body is designed to lose weight in the first 30 days following birth. Breastfeeding moms are often most aware of this initial weight loss. This is normal and natural so enjoy it.

The initial 5-6 weeks after having your baby is arguably the most exhausting. There are constant demands upon you and it is a time of great change and transition from life before motherhood to life now. Once you have recovered from this initial busy period, you will begin to feel that you have reached a greater physical and mental capacity and begin to desire more structured exercise. Some breastfeeding women find that they are no longer losing weight after the first 6-8 weeks. This is because the body has stabilized and got used to the excess calories that are being burned through feeding. Your body adapts and matches this demand by increasing calorie intake, thus negating the positive impact of breastfeeding for weight loss, and either stalling weight loss or even creating weight gain. If this has happened, or is happening to you, then it's a good time to reduce your calorie intake and start to exercise on a regular basis. Both these things will aid you in beginning to lose weight again.

Enjoy what you do!

As I have already said, I have met many people who aren't training for any particular event, yet they only partake in one form of exercise such as running or swimming. Some people even persevere with this one type of exercise despite the fact that they don't even enjoy it. I want to encourage you to try new things and to partake in a wide range of sports, classes, and activities. This keeps exercise fresh, challenging and rewarding as you continue to learn new skills, experience new places and meet new people. It helps avoid any possibility of boredom, which may lead to eventually quitting. I am not against choosing a sport or activity and sticking to it. There are benefits to this too. You see great improvement, you learn perseverance, and you achieve a much higher level in the chosen activity, experiencing great satisfaction! I am, however, trying to encourage those who are disillusioned with physical activity, those who seem to do the same old boring exercise, to try something new. I am sure everyone can find an activity that personally suits them and which they enjoy. Vary your activities, after all "variety is the spice of life". If you enjoy what you do, you are more likely to do it regularly and stick at it long enough to reap the benefits. If you enjoy exercising with others, do that. If you enjoy working out alone, do that. Discover your preference for being indoors or outdoors, being somewhere with music and noise or somewhere peaceful and tranquil. Find out what you enjoy and do it!

Progress, but progress slowly!

Please do not do the same session week in, week out without any change or progression. You will not be gaining the benefits you should be and you will soon become bored.

There is a principle in the science of training called "progressive overload" which was developed by Thomas Delorme, M.D. while he rehabilitated soldiers after World War II. He states that progressive overload is the gradual increase of stress placed upon the body during exercise training. Basically, in order to achieve more strength as opposed to maintaining the current strength capacity, the body's muscles must be overloaded. This overload stimulates the body's natural, adaptive processes to cope with the new demands placed on it. The adapted body is thus stronger than before the load had been placed on it.

I am a great believer in progressions. Once you have mastered one level in an exercise, and it begins to feel easier, your body has adapted and the muscles, tendons, ligaments and connective tissues are stronger, and you're ready to progress and move on to the next level. If there is no progression, there is no adaptation. Individuals who exercise sporadically never achieve any adaptation. They get the pains and aches after the initial session and then leave it so long before the next session that they never build on this. That means that whenever they return to exercise, they are always at the same level. They never lift any heavier, run any faster or ride any further.

Always start easy, and progress. Once you have successfully completed the first exercises, pain free and with good technique you are ready to move on to the next level, and not before. Pushing yourself too hard too soon could cause injury, discouragement and breakdown.

Free weights or weights machines?

Unless you have had an injury and are specifically carrying out rehab on a muscle or joint, you should stay away from weights machines and should lift dumbbells, kettle bells, barbells, sand bags or medicine balls. Machines work within a fixed plane of movement, making them excellent for early stages of rehab, and special situations, however for day-to-day training they are limited. The problem with machines is that they control the movement so that the body does not develop strength in multiple planes. This means that such movements do not prepare the body for real life situations. The muscles do not learn to balance and control the weights. In real life the body is required to absorb forces, control external loads and react to unpredictable movements. When the body is not prepared for this, it can end in injury.

Training with free weights and the types of implements listed above allows your body to develop this strength, balance, control, and coordination. The ability to receive accurate perceptual information about joint position and movement, and respond to this is called proprioception. Lifting with free weights trains your proprioception as well as your strength and so is much more realistic to real life.

Consistency

This is probably the number 1 rule for exercise. It very much reinforces my philosophy of a lifetime of fitness. Fitness is not about the occasional workout or an active day here and there, and it's certainly not some distant memory in the past! It is a lifestyle choice. A commitment to health and well-being that is fun and enjoyable. Thus, when it comes to getting fit, lots of little sessions on a regular basis over a period of weeks, months, and years are much more effective than a really hard session every now and then. That doesn't mean I am not a believer of hard work. Of course, it's good to push yourself, look for improvements and allow your body to adapt and get stronger and fitter. But it's good to remember that if you don't have the time for a long session, it's better to do something short than nothing at all. So many people think that since they don't have much time, they will wait and do a session when they have more time. This might be 3 or 4 days or even a week later. In that time, they could have done 4 or 5 short, intense 15-minute sessions which is much more effective than one long 1 or even 2-hour session! So, remember "Little and Often". A few lunges and squats can take just a few minutes!

Spot reduction is impossible!

The term spot reduction is used to suggest you can choose an area of your body and target that area for specific fat reduction. This is impossible. There is a lot of misinformation out there. There are people selling machines, which they claim to burn fat on your bum or your thighs or your tummy. ... The truth is, that none of these works. Let's have a look at why.

The bottom line is simple. You need to decrease body fat through dietary manipulation and exercise. The combination of reduced body fat and increased lean muscle mass leads to a more "toned" look.

What about Energy levels?

Your ability to exercise is dependent on your energy levels and your psychological state i.e. how you feel about exercising. Many people believe that if they feel they don't have the energy to exercise then they should not exercise. However, your felt energy levels can be affected by the amount of sleep you have had, the mood you are in, what you have eaten, your blood sugar levels, your caffeine intake and your level of desire for exercise. If you consistently get too little sleep, have one sugar spike or caffeine spike after the next, chances are you are very rarely going to feel like you have the energy to exercise. Sitting on the sofa with another cup of coffee and a chocolate bar seems far more appealing and feels like what your body needs, when actually; exercise is most likely exactly what your body needs! Exercising can actually be extremely energizing, and missing out on your exercise session could make you feel like you have even less energy!

To get a 'fair' and true reflection of your actual energy levels there are several areas to consider. You need to make sure you are getting to bed early to ensure as much sleep as possible when you have a new baby to care for during the night. Being sleep deprived will have a negative impact on your ability to exercise. You should be eating a diet with fewer sugar spikes, and not drinking too much caffeine. Both these factors can impact your desire to exercise and quality of exercise session. Both can mask how you are actually feeling in a positive or negative way. A sugar spike and the following low can make you feel tired and lethargic when actually you have plenty glycogen energy stores in your muscles and you are capable of a great exercise session and are ready to go!

Ssssssssssleep...

As you have read in my chapter titled Rest, Recovery and Sleep, sleep is extremely important in the post pregnancy period. Most people know that sleep is important for your health, but once you start adding exercise into your busy schedule, its importance increases.

It may be a difficult concept to understand but a good workout breaks down your body and it's the effective and adequate rest and sleep that follows that repairs it and makes it stronger. Therefore, no matter how hard you train, if you don't get sufficient sleep, you are compromising your recovery and subsequent training, and in effect wasting your time. The best results come when you work hard and rest well. During deep sleep, growth hormone production increases. It is this which helps to repair and rebuild muscles, and build strong bones after training. It is also worth noting that growth hormone production and release also promotes fat burning!

The National Sleep Foundation in the USA state that while naps cannot make up for inadequate night time sleep, a quick nap of 20-30 minutes may improve your mood, alertness and performance of tasks. Further research in a NASA study suggested that a 40-minute nap improved the performance of sleepy military pilots and astronauts by 34% and increased alertness by 100%. Therefore, I urge you to take a nap if the opportunity arises, especially if you have exercised. If it works for astronauts it works for moms!

Interestingly though, not only is sleep essential for rest and recovery, and for adaptation to exercise, but inversely, exercise is key to achieving good sleep. In fact, studies show that those struggling with insomnia should exercise more, and the more intense the exercise, the better the sleep that follows!

Exercise or Good Nutrition- Which is more important?

Exercise alone, is not the optimum source of weight loss. Exercise needs to be combined with a healthy eating plan in order to lose weight the best way. In fact, in some cases, people who exercise vigorously and regularly, yet have poor nutrition are unable to lose weight or achieve their desired body composition. On the other hand, there are individuals who look slim and fit, and perhaps have a good diet, however, they do not exercise, and therefore are not as healthy as they might look. Therefore, whatever your motivation for exercise, whether for health or body shape, or something else, you should realize that your exercise must be combined with good nutrition! You should not exercise solely to lose weight; after all, once you've achieved your ideal weight you won't need to lose any more. Be motivated by the fact that you are improving your health for you and your family, which in turn will allow you to live your life to the full!

Tips before you start

Keep in mind what your body has been through and don't expect too much too soon. Do not put yourself under unnecessary pressure to get fit overnight. Be realistic.

Good breast support is necessary. You should make sure you get a good support bra as your breasts will be larger than normal and if you are breastfeeding, they are also likely be tender. If you do not get the right support you may feel uncomfortable when you exercise.

You only need the bare minimum in terms of equipment. A set of gym clothes, a comfortable pair of trainers and a floor mat will be sufficient.

During each exercise session start slowly and increase your intensity gradually but steadily. This also applies to your exercise routine as a whole.

Be aware that after pregnancy your ligaments may be lax, leading to hyper-mobility, particularly round the hip and pelvic areas. Therefore, for the first few months do not work to extreme ranges of motion to avoid putting unnecessary pressure on your joints.

Drink regularly during and after exercise particularly if you are breastfeeding. Your body requires water for many of its vital functions.

Getting started

Getting started is one of the hardest things. Not just because of the lack of motivation, but more so due to the fact that many people do not know what to do to actually get started! Below is an outline, showing a safe and effective process from recovering from birth, to gentile exercise, to high level training for weight loss and gaining a great post pregnancy body.

Although realistically, much of a mom's motivation to exercise is to regain previous body shape, exercise should be stress-relieving not stress-provoking. The American Council on Exercise suggests that the goal of exercise after giving birth should be to help with relaxation, stress management, rehabilitation and emotional well-being rather than the goal of getting your previous body back.

When you initially try to do any kind of stomach exercises, you will very quickly realize that you simply can't. Your abdominal muscles have been stretched and, in most cases, pulled apart and no longer work! Don't panic. You are able to quickly re-learn how to use them and re-train them to work effectively by following the step-by-step progression of exercises that follow. This is a time in your life when you will need to do a lot of abdominal work to recover their position, heal and re-gain their strength. Once you have gone through this process, you will be able to maintain a strong core by doing very little isolated abdominal work and concentrating more on whole body movements (which also work your abs).

You should not feel that you need to slow down after having a baby. Of course, you will feel tired at times, especially during the first 4-6 weeks, that's normal, but you should be as active as you can be. Get plenty of rest when baby is sleeping and if you can, go to bed early. Remember, sleep helps heal the body and aids in recovery from exercise.

One of the biggest things on your mind is probably losing the weight you gained while you were pregnant. Remember that it took nine months to gain the weight, (which was distributed in a certain manner to support pregnancy and breastfeeding), and this weight gain did and does serve a purpose! Now, the process of losing this weight will take a similar amount of time. Be gentle with yourself, and give yourself the time to lose the weight in a healthy, positive way!

Post pregnancy return to exercise – The START of the program

Level 1 – Abdominal Breathing Exercises & Pelvic Floor Exercises

(Weeks 1-2)

The easiest way to get started with exercise is by doing Abdominal Breathing Exercises. These can be done as early as day 1. Although these exercises are not strenuous, the abdominal muscles can be strengthened through abdominal breathing, whilst the body relaxes. Lie flat on your back on the floor with your head supported by pillows. Gently place one hand on top of your abdomen and inhale deeply. As you inhale, the abdomen will rise higher. Hold this for five seconds, and then slowly release the air, watching the abdomen fall back to its original position. Hold this position for five seconds, repeating the process four to six times.

Pelvic floor exercises, called Kegel exercises after the gynecologist who created them, can and should be done within the first few days after birth. They require no gym membership, exercise mat or even a need to put aside time for this "exercise session". In fact, they can be done standing up, sitting down watching TV, waiting for the bus, or anywhere really – and no one will know you're doing them! Kegel exercises don't just strengthen the pelvic floor, but they also help support the abdomen similarly to the abdominal breathing exercises.

If you wish to lie down, lie flat on your back and bend your knees with your feet flat on the floor. Relax your head on the floor and look up at the ceiling. Contract the muscles of your vagina as if you are trying to stop the flow of urine. Make sure you are not just contracting your bum muscles. Hold this for 4-5 seconds. Repeat 10 times. Do 3-5 sets of this spaced throughout the day.

It's important to first build your pelvic floor muscles and deep core muscles through doing these exercises before you begin to work on your superficial abdominal muscles. Skipping this step will slow your progress and cause slow adaptation to another core work.

The Level 1 exercises can be carried on throughout Level 2 and Level 3 for as long as you feel necessary. In fact, by doing these pelvic floor exercises for 6-8 weeks, you will get an added benefit.

Level 2 – Early Progressions of Core Exercises

(Weeks 2-4)

The core is an important part of the body that acts as a support to all movements that the human body makes. It is the center of control and from it the arms and legs operate. To me, the core consists of more than just the abdominal muscles. The core consists of the whole mid-section of the body, which includes the abdominals, hips, pelvis, and lower back. The core plays an essential role in posture, which is vital for overall health and vitality. Moreover, posture is important for being able to execute exercises correctly.

Initially after birth, there is a gap in the abdominals that will take time to knit back together. It feels odd and there is the sensation that you have no strength in your abs at all. You are likely to be unable to perform simple tasks. Even sitting up to get out of bed may be a challenge, and you may find yourself having to first roll onto your side in order to get out of bed. These specific exercises have been chosen because they will help to close the gap that was formed during pregnancy, regain the strength and function of your abs, and enable you to get back to normal. You will even be able to use these alongside other exercises and methods to get a flat stomach and even a 6 pack if that's what you want!

Checklist

Make sure you perform each exercise with good form.

It's better to start with 3-5 repetitions done well, than 10 repetitions done poorly

Work up to 2-3 sets of 10 repetitions (except where otherwise stated)

Work through the range of motion that your body allows you to and progress towards working through a full range of motion. (Warning – during the first 6 weeks after birth DO NOT push your ligaments to their maximum capacity – see earlier in chapter)

Think about breathing in during the easy part of the movement and breathing out at the end of the effort.

Remember "form, posture, breathing"

When you have mastered all of the core exercises in Level 2, move on to Level 3 but not before.

Seated isometric Abs squeezes

Try sitting up tall and squeezing your belly inwards to your spine. Start with 20 each day, working up to 100 each day.

Pelvic tilts

Stand straight with your back to the wall and relax your spine. Breathing in deeply, and press the small of your back against the wall. Exhale and repeat. Continue the exercise for 1-2 minutes. These can be repeated several times throughout the day.

Happy cat, angry cat

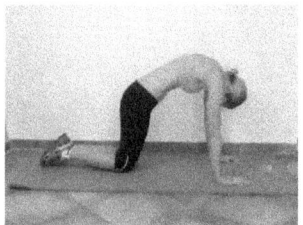

Kneel on all fours and round your back with your head pointing downwards. Tilt your pelvis forwards.

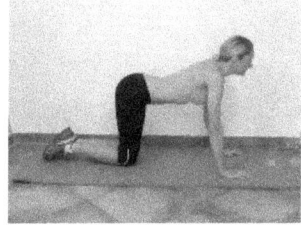

Slowly transition to an arched back position with your head looking upwards and your pelvis tilted backwards.

Single arm drop

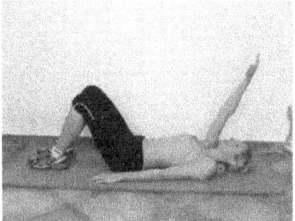

Lie flat on your back with your arms by your side, head looking upwards and spine neutral. Bend your knees and put your heels on the floor. Raise one arm upwards and above your head. Move your arm slowly backwards and forwards whilst maintaining your neutral spine position (there should be no movement in your back).

Single leg drops

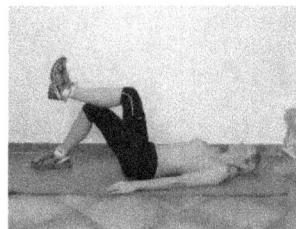

Lie flat on your back with your arms by your side, head looking upwards and spine neutral. Bend your knees and put your heels on the floor. Raise one knee upwards towards your chest, and then back to its resting position.

Double leg hip bridge

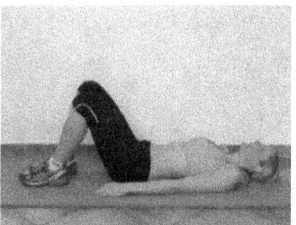

Lie flat on your back with your arms by your side, head looking upwards and spine neutral. Bend your knees and put your feet flat on the floor.

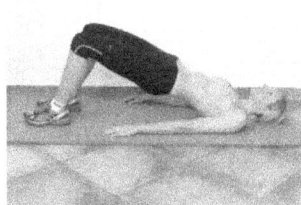

Pushing your feet into the floor and squeezing your glutes (buttocks), raise your hips upwards until you achieve a straight line from your knees to your shoulders. Return to the start position and repeat this.

Fire Hydrants

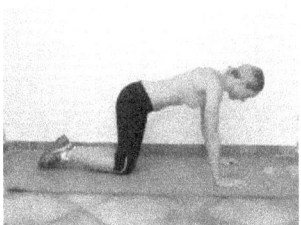

Kneel on all fours, and hold your tummy in whilst maintaining a flat back. Keep your head in a neutral position.

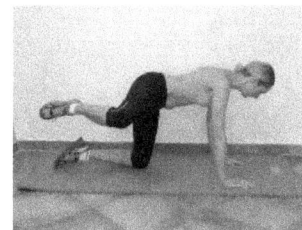

Slowly lift one leg out sideways and then back to the start position whilst maintaining a neutral spine and head position throughout.

4-point kneeling arm raise

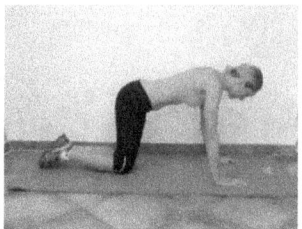

Kneel on all fours, and hold your tummy in whilst maintaining a flat back. Keep your head in a neutral position.

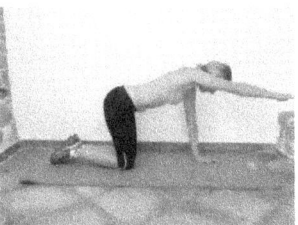

Slowly lift one arm out in front then place it back to the floor. Maintain a neutral spine and head position throughout.

4-point kneeling leg raise

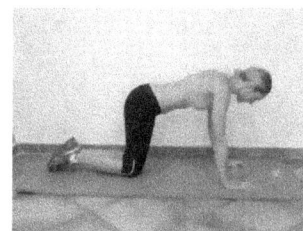

Kneel on all fours, and pull your tummy in, maintaining a flat back. Keep your head in a neutral position.

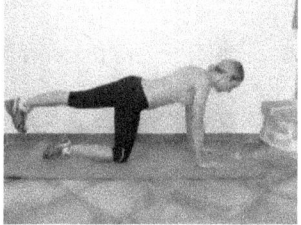

Slowly lift one leg out behind then place it back to the floor. Maintain a neutral spine and head position throughout.

Clams

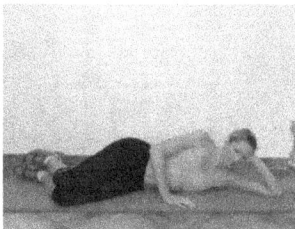

Lie on your side with your head supported in your hand and bend both legs comfortably underneath you.

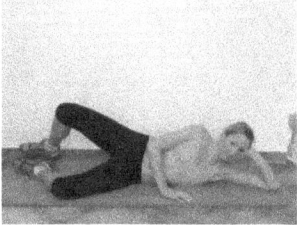

Slowly lift your knee upwards, initiating the movement from your glutes whilst keeping your hips in the same position.

Side lying knee lift

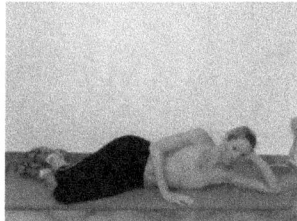

Lie on your side with your head supported in your hand and bend both legs comfortably underneath you.

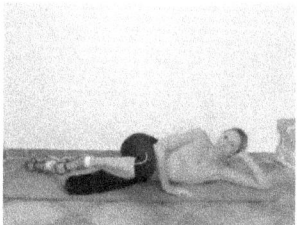

Bring the knee of your top leg upwards towards your chest then back to a straight position in line with your body.

Knee lift & kickbacks

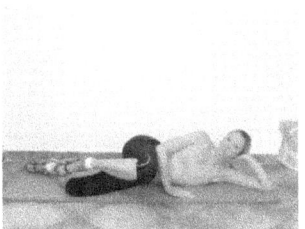

Lie on your side with your head supported in your hand and bend both legs comfortably underneath you. Bring the knee of your top leg upwards towards your chest.

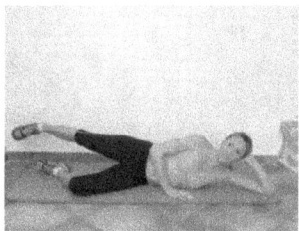

Extend the leg backwards and kick out behind you whilst maintaining your body posture.

Heel touch

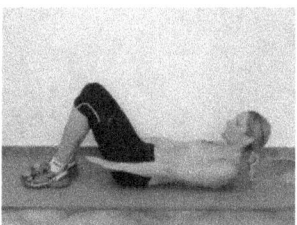

Lie on your back with your knees bent, heels flat on the floor, and arms by your side. Crunch upwards, slightly raising your shoulders off the mat.

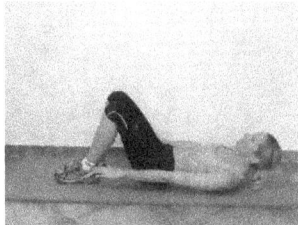

Move side-to-side moving your hand towards your heel, without letting your shoulders touch the mat.

Single leg fallouts

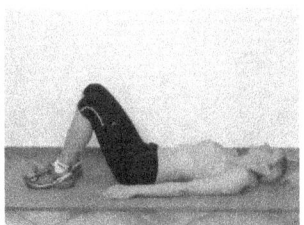

Lie flat on your back with your arms by your side. Keep your head looking upwards and spine neutral. Bend your knees and lift one foot off the floor binging the knee towards the chest.

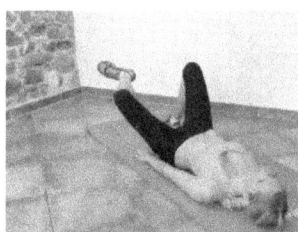

Allow the leg which is off the floor to fallout to one side through movement of the hip joint, and then bring this knee back to the start position.

Hip drops

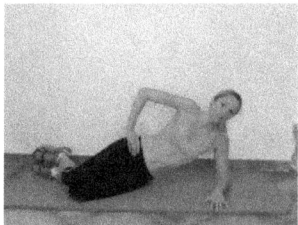

Lie on your side with your elbow and knees on the floor and one hand on your hip.

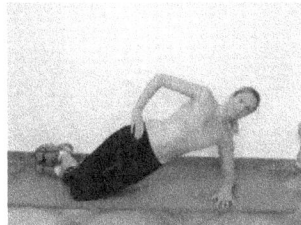

Lift your hips upwards to the position where your body is in a straight line and lower your hips down again. Do this repeatedly.

Half side planks

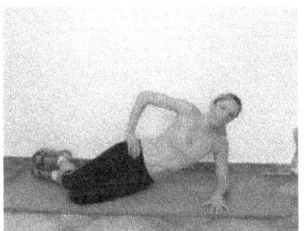

Lie on your side with your elbow and knees on the floor and one hand on your hip.

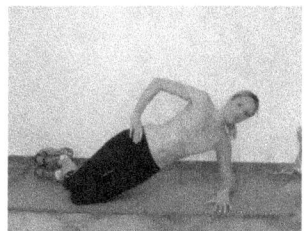

Lift your hips upwards to the position where your body is in a straight line and hold this position until you begin to lose form. Work up to 1 minute.

Level 3 – Further Progressions of Core Exercises

(Weeks 4-6)

The following exercises are progressions of the earlier exercises shown in Level 2. They are more difficult to perform. If you cannot perform Level 2 exercises correctly, you will not be able to perform the following ones with good form. As a result, you will be putting your body at risk of injury. Only when you are able to perform 2-3 sets of 10+ repetitions of the Level 2 exercises with no pain and with perfect form, are you ready to move onto the further progressions of the core exercises.

The exercises in Level 3 follow the same principles as the ones above. Progress slowly from 3-5 repetitions until you can perform 2-3 sets of 10 repetitions (except where otherwise stated). Ensure good form for each repetition, in order not to put your body at risk of injury.

Double bent leg lift

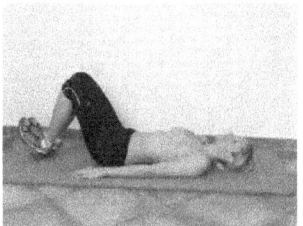

Lie flat on your back with your arms by your side, head looking upwards and spine neutral. Bend your knees and put your heels on the floor.

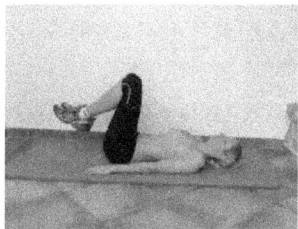

Slowly raise your knees upwards towards your chest whilst maintaining a flat back. Draw your abs in whilst maintaining relaxation throughout the rest of your body.

Single Straight leg lift

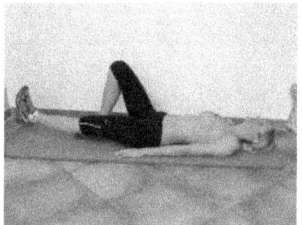

Lie flat on your back with your arms by your side, head looking upwards and spine neutral. Bend one leg and keep the other leg straight.

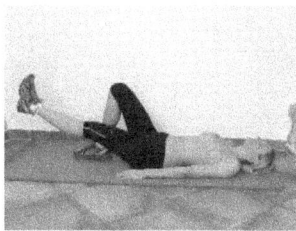

Slowly lift the straight leg off the floor. Initially use your hands to help by pushing into the floor. Progress this by turning your palms upwards and not using your hands to push. Maintain a neutral spine throughout the movement.

Leg bounces at 90°

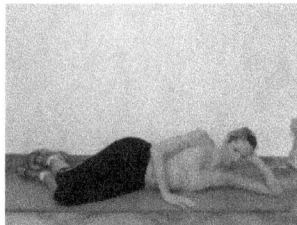

Lie on your side with your head supported in one hand and the other hand on the floor in front of you for support.

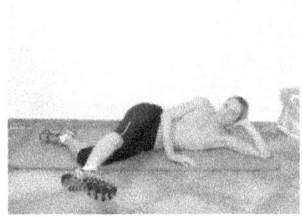

Extend your top leg out in front at 90° and bounce up and down with small movements for 30 seconds

Opposite Arm and leg lifts

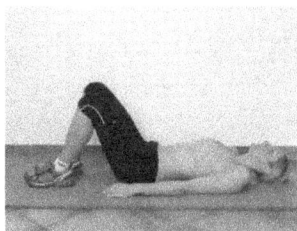

Lie flat on your back with your arms by your side, head looking upwards and spine neutral. Bend your knees and put your feet flat on the floor.

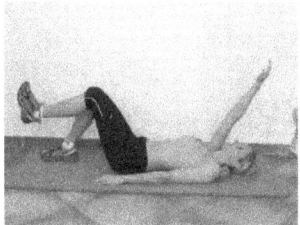

Lift one arm and the opposite leg. As you lower your leg, lower your arm. Repeat with the other arm and leg.

Dead bugs

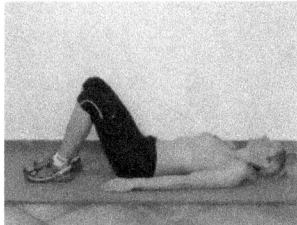

Lie flat on your back with your arms by your side, head looking upwards and spine neutral. Bend your knees and put your feet flat on the floor.

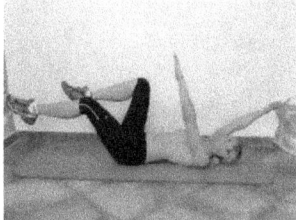

Lift one arm and the opposite leg. Stretch your arm above your head and lower the opposite leg to the floor simultaneously. Repeat with the other arm and leg so that both arms and legs are moving simultaneously in opposite directions.

Front plank

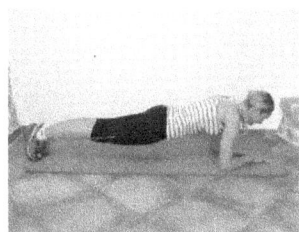

Hold your body as flat as possible with your weight on your forearms and toes. Maintain a straight line through your body with your head in a neutral position. Hold still for as long as you can until you lose form. Work up to 1 minute.

Crunch

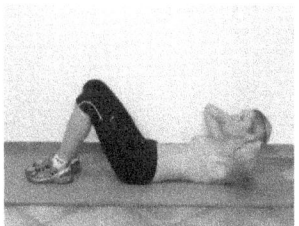

Lie flat on your back with your knees bent and feet flat on the floor. Place your hands behind your head for support. Slowly crunch upwards by raising your shoulders off the mat. Return slowly to the start position.

Single leg hip bridge

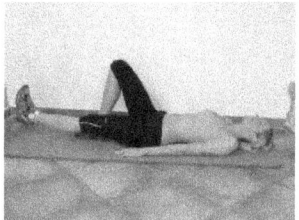

Lie flat on your back with your arms by your side, head looking upwards and spine neutral. Bend one knee and keep the other leg straight.

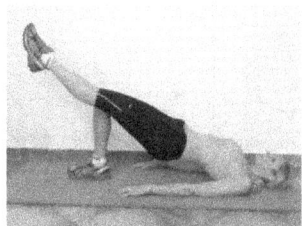

Pushing your foot into the floor and squeezing your glutes (buttocks), raise your hips and leg upwards until you achieve a straight line from the toe of your extended leg to your shoulders. Lower your hips back down to the mat to return to the start position. Work up to 10 repetitions. Repeat on the same number with the opposite leg.

4-point kneeling, opposite arm and leg raise

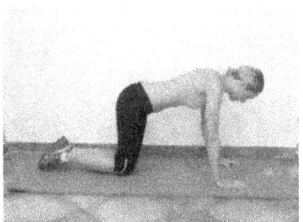

Kneel on all fours, hold your tummy in maintaining a flat back and keep your head in a neutral position.

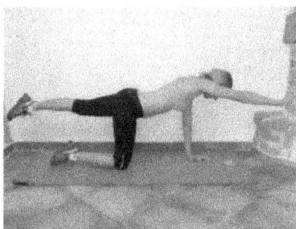

Slowly and simultaneously lift one arm out in front, and the opposite leg out behind then place them back to the floor. Repeat on the other side. Maintain a neutral spine and head position throughout the movement.

Half side plank with leg lift

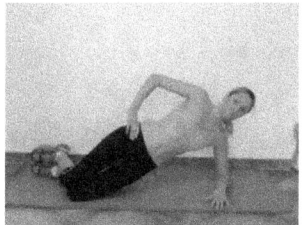

Hold the half side plank position described in Level 2, with your weight on your knees and forearm.

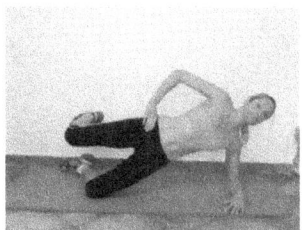

Either raise your knee up and down whilst maintaining a strong core, or raise your knee upwards and hold this position for as long as you can without losing form.

Side plank

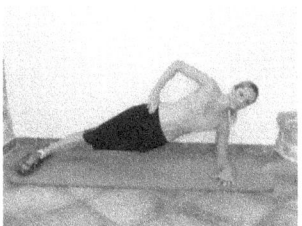

Lie on your side then raise your weight off the mat so that all your weight rests on your forearm and feet. For balance, place the foot of your top leg in front of the foot of your back leg.

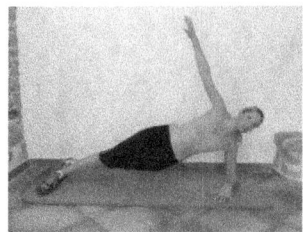

Vary this by either raising your hand into the air, or by raising one leg up like in the half side plank above.

During week 4-6, whilst you are doing Level 3, you should aim to swim or walk regularly in addition to performing the core exercises. Both swimming and walking provide muscle toning, low impact workouts. The heart and lungs benefit too. Swimming, however, may have to wait until you stop secreting lochia. As soon as the discharge finishes, you're ready to go.

Level 4 – Full-body Conditioning, Jogging, & Cycling

(Weeks 6-10)

As you progress through the first 3 levels and can feel your body getting stronger and fitter, you are ready to continue further to full-body conditioning exercises, jogging and cycling. As you begin to increase the intensity and duration, you can begin to play some sport again or take part in more rigorous exercise. I have encouraged waiting until this point to start sport or vigorous forms of exercise again.

This is due to the fact that until now, your ligaments have been lax and your body has not been used to the extreme range of movements and the speed of these movements, and so could easily get injured. Rebuilding a strong base first means that you are more likely to stay injury free and enjoy training problem free.

The overall plan at this point is to get into full body workouts and other activities such as sports, aerobic classes, or strength programs. These exercises in your workouts should be based round functional movements that apply to daily life.

Lifting weights will improve your strength and functional ability to perform daily tasks. Performed with correct technique it also protects your joints and can reduce back pain. I therefore like to recommend some form of weight training.

Progress from core/floor work to full body conditioning! Here are some excellent exercises that I like to include at different times in a training program:

Push-ups with knees on the floor or push-ups with feet on the floor

Other pushing exercises like bench press and push press (varying between bar and dumbbells)

Pull-ups with bands to aid

Other pulling exercises like horizontal pulls to a bar and bent over row

Squatting, including wide sumo style squats and single leg squats

Overhead squats (bar above the head)

Step-ups (onto a bench or step with dumbbells or a barbell)

Lunges (forwards and backwards)

Lateral lunges

Arabesque (Single leg "good morning" or Single leg Romanian dead lift)

Romanian dead lift

These exercises should first be mastered using your body weight and being performed for 3 sets of 10-12 repetitions without loss of form. Once this can be done well, you can add weight to these and see yourself progress. If these exercises are new to you and you want to use weights, I recommend learning them under the supervision of a Personal Trainer or Coach. Otherwise you may not be doing them correctly and could be putting yourself at risk of injury.

Level 5 – Strength Training & all forms of Sport

(Weeks 8-12 and onwards) Yippee!!!

Once you reach this stage you have laid an excellent foundation through progressing your exercises and abilities over an 8 to 10-week period. You are now ready to progress to higher intensity exercises or exercise classes, weight training, interval training or sports.

There are so many different sports and activities that you can enjoy to keep fit. I'm hoping that through your journey back to fitness after having your baby, or perhaps your journey to fitness for the first time, you have felt inspired to try something different. This could be buying a new exercise DVD that involves exercises that you have never done before. It could be taking up a new sport, or joining a new club or class. You may decide to take up CrossFit, or train for a 5K race, a triathlon, or maybe a half marathon or even marathon! You may, like me, chose to do a mixture of activities. I enjoy weight training, exercise DVDs, circuit-style training, Zumba, skiing, roller blading, cycling, swimming, tennis and occasional jogging (!). The opportunities are vast.

You may have met new people or made new friends through attending exercise classes, or through going to the gym. Whatever has changed for you going through this process, I want to encourage you to stay active, fit and healthy.

Stretching

Stretching is an important form of exercise, especially after a workout. If you spend a small amount of time stretching each major muscle group that you have used in the exercise session, it will help your recovery. Stretching relaxes the muscles and helps realign the muscle fibers, causing them to return to their pre-exercise state. If you find it hard to stretch regularly, or don't really know the best way to do it, you may benefit from a Yoga class, as this is a great way of stretching. Stretching is also good for maintaining and improving flexibility, which is an important aspect of health and fitness. As we age, we lose flexibility in our muscles and joints, and therefore are at greater risk of injury. By maintaining, or improving flexibility, we are reducing our risk of injury and extending our functional physical ability i.e. our ability to perform daily tasks.

Breastfeed your baby

It is a lot of work having an infant sucking milk from your breast. Many women do not realize this. As the infant is getting the needed nutrients and vitamins, the mother also gains by losing the baby weight because breast-feeding makes a woman's uterus shrink back to its original size thus very crucial in losing baby weight. In addition, breastfeeding, done over six months, burns around four hundred calories per day! Not bad eh! Ignore the naysayers that tell you that dieting and exercise dry up breast milk. There is no relation between dieting and quantity of breast milk a woman produces. If you cannot breastfeed, it is okay, try other options instead. Ignore those people that tell you that you are a bad mother because you do not breastfeed. People with most closed minds have the most open mouths!

Think slim
Avoid fatty foods. Sit at the table to eat, not at the TV Resist the urge to get second helpings. It is best to avoid high fat comfort foods to make you feel better when you are under stress. Try relaxation methods instead. Eat at least five portions of fruits and vegetables for a faster metabolism.

Snacking as part of healthy eating

Consumption of excessive sugar drastically increases your blood-sugar levels. When the level of your blood sugar drops back to normal, you are more prone to consume the first food you see. So, wage an immortal war on the sugary treats. Keep away from temptation by storing only nutritious foods at your side. Eating healthy snacks is crucial to baby weight loss. It allows you to eat between meals without worrying about weight gain. Choose low fat foods to snack on such as fruits, vegetables, and slimmer's soup. Eating snacks high in fiber similar to crackers or figs and raisins, makes you feel full so you will not need a second helping. Here is an example of a good snack that is just fifty calories:

1 cup slimmer's soup
1-cup low calorie chocolate drink
1 biscotti
1-amaretto biscuit
Vegetables with 1 tbsp. Low fat soft cheese or 2 tbsp. salsa

Find other new moms interested in baby weight loss.
It helps a great deal if you can find other moms that want to lose baby weight. Many new moms agree that exercising with a group is much more effective than doing it all by yourself. So, what are waiting for? Get yourself in a group today!

Hydrate!
When we are thirsty, we often interpret as being hungry so most likely we will eat. If you drink enough water, you will hardly feel thirsty or hungry because the water will fill you up. This is way much easier and more effective than going to the gym, risk opening your abdominal stitches (if you had C.S).

Cheat Mother Nature
If you cut back on what you eat, you give the body the impression of scarcity. This is counterproductive, as the body will turn even the littlest amount of food into fat! Cheat nature by eating five small meals in a day to give the impression of abidance of food. You will lose the baby weight in no time!

Napping

Sleep well. Studies show that those who were sleep deprived gain weight than those who had good sleep. Yes, the baby may interfere with your sleep, but when the baby sleeps, you sleep, forget the chores. You owe this to yourself.

When you sleep well, you have energy; you are not tempted to eat high calorie food substances to regain energy. This is crucial in baby weight loss.

In all, relax, take a break you will lose the weight!

Nutrition is Key

Prior to beginning any new diet regime, please consult with your doctor, and be weary of your recommended daily caloric intake. Please note: If you are breastfeeding, your caloric intake will be higher per your doctor's specified advice.

Similar to a car, our bodies need fuel; and the kind of fuel we put in our tanks gives us different results in performance. I'm not a mechanic, but I have rescued a few friends on the side of the road, due to their cars running out of gas or breaking down etc. Cars and fuel work as a metaphor, because this is all true of our human bodies as well. If we eat junk, our bodies turn into junk, and our minds cannot focus; which creates an endless cycle of tiredness and no progression whatsoever. Our bodies cannot perform without the proper nutrition; aka fuel.

We must return to basic, healthy food groups; and most importantly- repeat after me: ADDED SUGAR IS EVIL AND TOXIC. Jumping back to the car metaphor: Do you know what happens if someone pours a bag of sugar in your car's gas tank? Answer: your car would die, and never run again. This is true, just ask your mechanic. Added Sugar will do the same to our human bodies as it does to our cars: kills our performance and potential. So sorry if that scares you, but it is the truth. On that note, let's start off nutrition with the most important lesson in Losing the Baby Weight: ADDED SUGAR IS EVIL AND TOXIC.

Natural Sugar versus Added Sugar

Fruits, veggies, and other plant derived foods have natural sugar; this is different than "Added Sugar." Natural sugars are easily broken down by the body, but only as nature intended: in small doses. Some would say Cane Sugar is natural, but let me explain an important fact as to why it boils down to how things are processed. For instance, granulated sugar is processed from a plant, called Sugar Cane. Most people know this, but not many people consider how much Sugar Cane Plant it takes to make 1 pound of granulated sugar. Do you know how granulated sugar is processed? Below is an illustration diagram on how the sugar cane plant is processed into granulated sugar.

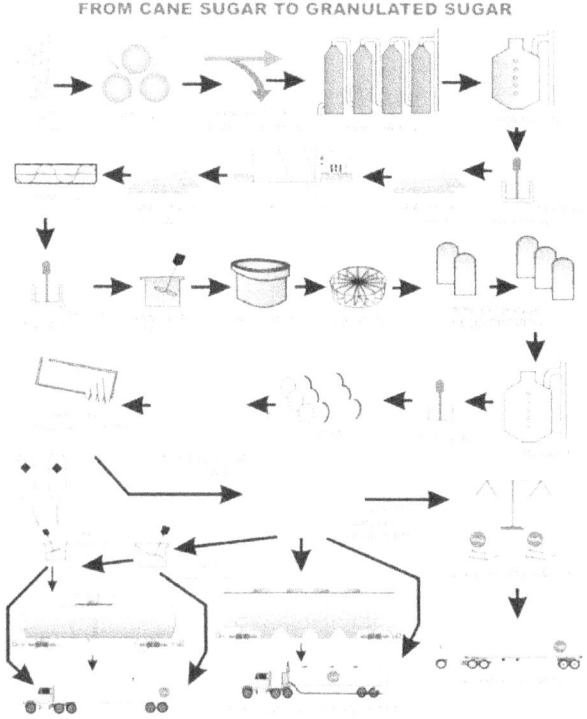

FROM CANE SUGAR TO GRANULATED SUGAR

Crazy, isn't it? Even if they stopped at Raw Sugar, the 6th step in the process, and skipped so much of the other chemical break-down, our bodies are not built to consume so many Sugar Cane Plants in one sitting. In other words, let's break it down to simple sugar math.

Simple Sugar Math

1. An average sugarcane stalk weighs about 3 pounds (1.3 kilograms) and is 85% juice. How many pounds of juice will an average stalk produce?

Answer: 2.6 pounds (1.1 kilograms) of juice.

2. The juice squeezed out of a sugarcane stalk is about 11% sugar by weight. How many pounds of sugar can be produced from one stalk?

Answer: An average stalk contains about 0.3 pounds (0.12 kilograms) of sugar.

3. How many stalks of sugarcane will it take to produce a 5-pound bag of sugar?

Answer: 16.67 canes are needed to make 5 pounds of granulated sugar. (Roughly 50 pounds of sugarcane stalks to make 5 pounds of granulated sugar.)

In 2015, the average American consumed 66.6 pounds of refined sugar, 62 pounds of corn-derived sweeteners, 1.5 pounds of honey and edible syrups, for a total caloric-sweetener annual consumption of 154.8 pounds. Yikes! All stats were found on FAITC.org (US Agriculture School Statistics.)

I know it is hard to follow because we are talking about sugar here! Let me break it down another way, because one truly needs to understand this in order to succeed in losing the baby weight. How would you feel after eating 1 orange versus 10 oranges? I think most people would have a tummy ache if they consumed 10 oranges in one sitting. Sugar Cane Stalk is a plant as well; therefore, if we look at it unprocessed, in its original state, and tried to eat it -one would look at Added Sugar very differently.

Coca cola that is made from cane sugar (not corn sugar) has roughly 1 processed stalk of sugar cane worth of Added Sugar. It's tough to compute why this is so horrible, but follow me on this important mindset change. Going back to the oranges, it is not nature's intention for us to eat 10 oranges in one sitting; just as it is not natural for us to eat a 3-pound stalk of Sugar Cane.

If you ever ate honeysuckle as a kid, it would take hundreds of honeysuckle flowers to make a teaspoon of juice. Same with Sugar Cane: only 11% of the juice extracted from the 3-pound stalk is processed into granulated sugar (roughly 39 grams or 10 teaspoons of Added Sugar.)

Our bodies can break down small doses of Added Sugar in a day, but no more than 20 grams before our liver gets overloaded (like a traffic jam on the freeway.) 20 grams is not very much compared to how much a normal person consumes of Added Sugar. To put in perspective, an average person consumes 76 grams of added sugar per day.

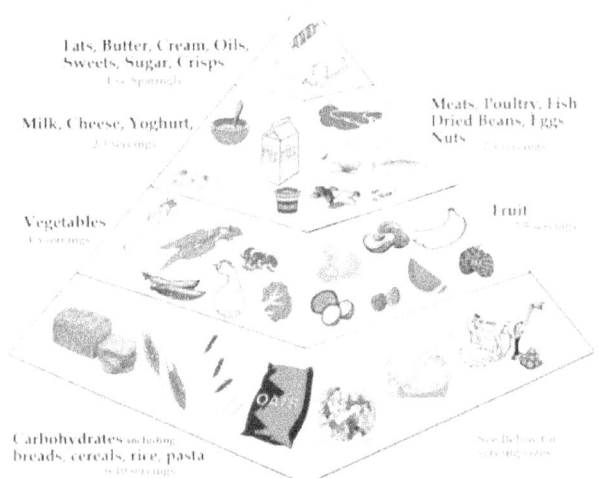

Conclusion

Ultimately, keeping in mind the power of good support and a mentally healthy mindset, you will lose the baby weight. Anybody who has the motivation to return to their pre-pregnancy body and has any discipline at all should be able to succeed. Nothing that I've discussed here is particularly groundbreaking or earth shattering. I also don't want anybody to think that I, like many of the quick-fix fads, am pushing some specific program and the only means of success. There are many different avenues one can take to succeed in slimming down after childbirth. There are, however, some fundamental truths including eating well, but not going on a crazy fad diet, and exercising, even if it means doing so in incremental and practical ways. I don't have all the answers, but I do know what worked for me. In the end, there will be no chance of achieving your goals if you don't put in a little bit of work. Nobody said it would be easy. Do the work, stay the course, overcome obstacles, and remain positive.